Ex-Acute 2017

Ex-Acute 2017

A Former Hospital CEO
Tells All on What's Wrong
With American Healthcare

Josh Luke

Library of Congress Control Number:		2016903095
ISBN:	Hardcover	978-1-5144-7003-9
	Softcover	978-1-5144-7004-6
	eBook	978-1-5144-7005-3

Printed in the USA

Rev. date: 01/31/2017

To order additional copies of this book, contact:
Xlibris
1-888-795-4274
www.Xlibris.com
Orders@Xlibris.com
736449

DEDICATION

I dedicate this book to my two beloved grandmothers who were both such inspirations to me. Both Belva Mae Riddle and Wanda Belle Gerken penned many personal letters to me in their lifetimes, a copy of one letter from each is included in this book. The first letter, written by Grandma Wanda to me on my eighteenth birthday in 1990, is on the page following this dedication. The second, from Grandma Belva is included later on in this this book, when I am speaking of her particular experiences with hospitalization and post-acute care. I am confident that each would be comfortable with me sharing their stories of aging, as they were both consistent in encouraging me to use my gifts, specifically writing. The confidence in me that both had expressed has brought me great strength, continuing to the present day. Enjoy. I know they both would. Miss you both dearly.

Dear Josh,

Cinco de Mayo, 1990, and you are eighteen, my youngest grandson
a voting adult! It doesn't seem possible that it can happen so
fast; It was such a short time ago that you were that curly-
headed little tyke with the great smile. Of course you still
have the smile, but you have done a lot of growing UP.

We have so enjoyed you, Josh, through your wild ideas and
schemes, your school activities, and in all of your sporting
events. You haven't had as much time to spend with us as we would
have liked but we hope one day your time won't be scheduled so
tightly and we will have that opportunity. We like having you
around, and you know you are welcome anytime. You have a great
sense of humor, and a smile that is always at the ready.

I can remember one day, waiting beside your crib, praying as hard
as I knew how, waiting for you to come out of a coma caused by a
Staph infection following one of your surgeries. Dr. Visut and
the nurses were in and out, trying anything they thought might save
you, finally using an experimental procedure that brought you back
to us. You slowly opened your eyes, and when you saw Grandpa and
me you gave us a big smile...as ill as you were you still had a smile.

And years later, when you sat on the bench, knowing you were as good
or even better than the guys on the court, you still had a pat on
the back and a smile for them when they came out. A great attitude!

Keep your faith strong, Josh. I think God must be a very good sport,
because He watches over us even though we ignore Him; However, if
you remember to thank Him for your daily blessings of family, friends,
safe passage through the day, and the little things we take for granted,
and also go to Him with your problems and your dreams and ambitions
you just can't imagine how much help you will get.

Josh, you really had a wide smile when you won the MVP trophy at the
basketball tournament, even though you were smiling through your
tears, and ours. That was one of the most exciting moments of our
life.....we almost burst with pride.

You have so much talent, and talent is a challenge and a responsibility as well as a gift. Use it. Never let it lay dormant. Even
though your profession is in another field don't stop expressing
yourself through poetry and the written word. You have already
written some very good material and I'm sure you have the potential
for even greater things.

If I sound a little prejudiced in your behalf maybe I am, but as
your very proud Grandmother I have that right. You have given us
every reason to be proud. We love you, and we want you to know
we are here for you. Have a great eighteenth birthday and a really
wonderful life.

Much love always,
Grandma Gerken

XXXXXXXXXXXXXXXXXXX0000000000000000000XXXXXXXXXXXXXXXXXX0000000000000
0000000000000000000XXXXXXXXXXXXXXXXXXXXX00000000000000000000XXXXXXXXXX

CONTENTS

Part 2: Lessons from the Field: Accessing Care for Your Aging Parents, Your family and Your Children

ACKNOWLEDGMENTS

Where to start?

Thanks to my wife for supporting me and teaching me that seasons of life are a real thing. She taught me early on that life is about understanding where you are in a storm cycle. As individuals, we are always in one of the following three categories:

- Preparing for a storm
- In the middle of a storm
- Or in between storms

Though I consider myself an optimist, her storm theory has become ingrained in me. I think it is an admirable approach to being prepared for what life throws at you and for not being stunned when caught off guard. I am grateful for her support through the travels, late nights on the computer, and changing of jobs that led to the career path which has shaped my unique experiences and philosophies. I am thankful to her for so much more, but in this season of life, the storm philosophy has proven to have better prepared us for unforeseen challenges.

I would also like to thank my editor, Shawn Noetzli. She edited not only this book but also my first book, Readmission Prevention: *Solutions across the Provider Continuum,* which was the best-selling health care book of 2015 for the American College of Healthcare Executives. Her editing expertise and knack for marketing and creating a powerful social media presence are second to none.

Also, I am grateful to Carissa Gaborow of CareCentrix for suggesting that the book title be "Ex-Acute 2017." Seeing that I am a former acute hospital CEO, when Carissa first suggested this, the others in the room laughed hysterically and thought it was a perfect fit for my "tell it how I see it" approach to health care. From that day forward,

I felt strongly that the "Ex-Acute 2017" title has a strong impact that I hope to convey with the words and stories in the book as well. Special thanks as well to Elizabeth Keough for inviting me to join Dr. Eric Coleman and Dr. Steven Jencks, two of the pioneers in the care transitions space, to share our expertise with CareCentrix's executives and Scientific Advisory Board in 2014.

Thanks to Xlibris Publishing for having the confidence in me to publish and market this book nationally and internationally. I am also proud to represent the Sol Price School of Public Policy at the University of Southern California and for the confidence that Dean Jack H. Knott, Mike Nichol (interim vice dean for faculty affairs), and Lavonna B. Lewis (teaching professor) have shown in me.

There are so many others to thank. Just know that you are all appreciated.

FOREWORD

Josh Luke has put on paper the thoughts and feelings of so many of us in the health care industry in a concise, articulate, and accessible format. He has decades of industry experience and has the sadly all-too-unique perspective of putting consumers first in every equation. Called by many the "Tony Robbins of Healthcare" as his presentations worldwide are equally educational, inspirational, and informative, Josh brings a real-world, boots-on-the-ground perspective not just of the hospital world but of the post-acute sector as well.

I met Josh many years ago and have been greatly impressed, watching him rise through the ranks of hospital administration and as he became one of the nation's foremost authorities on health care systems. Josh's passion for his work is only one way he has been dedicated to giving back to the world around him. His generosity of spirit is showcased through his gracious donation of literally tens of thousands of dollars to support people with dementia. That generosity stems not only from his family's personal journey but also from his character as a father, husband, and community leader.

This book speaks to the parent raising young children. It speaks to the adult children who are managing care for their aging parents. It speaks to everyone on their own level. I know you will enjoy this candid and direct take on the health care system as much as I did. His bold an accurate predictions over the last five years, in the face of many skeptics I might add, have almost all come to fruition and he has truly become 'The Voice of American Healthcare.'

Jim McAleer
Chief Executive Officer
Alzheimer's Orange County

PREFACE

I was fortunate enough to become the Chief Executive Officer of a hospital at age 32. Along the way, I questioned everything. You see, in spite of my prior training, I was still very much learning on the job. There were so many questions to be asked.

While my family has always been my priority, as my children grew into their teens I found myself asking the same question on a regular basis: Will my children be able to access healthcare as they grow older? I wished I could answer this question, but for many years I was unable.

Then at some point in 2015, someone suggested I share my experiences in healthcare with mainstream America in the form of a book, as a guide if you will, to assist individuals in navigating through America's complicated and expensive delivery system. As I thought about the suggestion to pen a book for mainstream America (I had already published a book for health care executives), I realized that if I do not have the answers to accessing health care in the future, who would? So I set out to create a book that could serve as a guide for adult children caring for aging parents, parents of young children, and any American interested in understanding our delivery system.

Thus, after more than fifteen years of managing hospitals and nursing homes, I prepared this manuscript. Part 1 of the book outlines the incentives and motivations of America's health care delivery system. The reader will gain a basic understanding of America's inefficient delivery model and why their personal doctor may not always be financially incentivized to be truthful to them. Part 2 is a guide for navigating and accessing health care in the model of the future—and it may save you a few bucks in the long run as well.

Enjoy this journey through recent health care history and the guide on how to best navigate the confusing delivery model as our country integrates a new delivery system.

PART 1

The Fee-for-Service
Merry-Go-Round

CHAPTER 1

Home Runs and Health Care:
How I Became a Hospital
CEO at Age Thirty-two

B LAME MY GRANDMOTHER for my passionate positions on health care delivery.

When I completed graduate school with a master's degree in public relations in 1996, my dream was to have a career in sports marketing. I grew up a huge sports fan, a junkie if you will, playing three sports in high school and scrumming it up in the front yard with my two older brothers, Scott and Matt, on a daily basis. The shape or size of the ball did not matter. While God blessed my two older brothers with much more athletic ability than me, I share my brothers' love for just about every sport.

Looking back, it was in 1998 that important milestones began to occur in my life. My brother Matt, who is just a year older than me, made it to the major leagues as a member of the Los Angeles Dodgers. It was that same year that I married my beautiful wife, Martine, and just a few months after my twenty-sixth birthday, I achieved what I believed to be my career goal up to that point of working in sports marketing. Through hard work and a stroke of good luck, just a few days after renowned baseball slugger Mark McGwire had broken the single-season home run record of sixty-one home runs in September 1998, the global public relations firm I was working for was retained to handle the new home run king's personal marketing and public relations. I was appointed the account lead. It was an exciting year indeed!

Just a few weeks after being hired to work with Mark McGwire, I found myself on a private jet, along with my newlywed wife, Martine, heading to New York with baseball's new home run king and some of his closest friends. The following day, I escorted Mark to interviews with *Time* magazine, who was considering him as a "Man of the Year" candidate; the *Today Show*; the *Late Show with David Letterman*; and the once-popular *Rosie O'Donnell Show*. It was the experience of a lifetime.

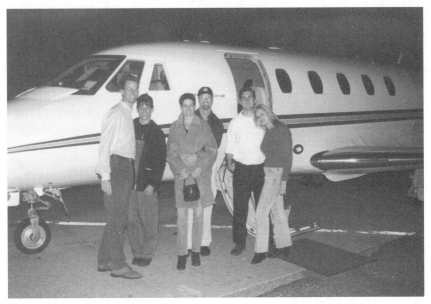

This trip on a private jet to New York in October 1998 proved to be both a highlight and a turning point in my career.

No doubt 1998 was an eventful year. However, it was what happened in the years that followed that really changed my life. Within a few years of our private jet trip to New York with one of the most recognizable faces in the world at that time, I found myself sharing with my wife that after working with professional athletes in golf, basketball, baseball, football, and hockey and having been exposed to almost every major sport, I was beginning to feel unfulfilled in my career. I was losing my love for professional sports by working so closely with athletes. It just felt to me like my chosen profession was irrelevant in the big picture now that I was married and more focused on raising a family. I felt like I wanted to make a greater impact on the world around me. It was at that same time that my beloved grandmother Belva Mae Riddle started to bounce back and forth between the hospital, the nursing home, and her home over what seemed like several years. Although my grandmother had a beautiful mind and was one of the most caring and strongest-willed individuals you would ever meet, her congestive heart failure started to progress at a rate that proved to be too much for her to handle by the summer of 2002.

While I was living outside of California at the time, completing my graduate studies, my frequent calls home to check on my grandmother often led to frustration. I was perplexed by how her caretakers at the hospital and in the nursing home had so little communication when she transferred from one facility to the other. I was even more shocked to find that when my grandma was transferred home from one of these facilities, the home-based caretakers seemed to have little instructional communication from the hospital or nursing home. How could this be possible? Was this the norm? How could they even care for my grandmother for a single hour without having up-to-the-minute notes from the nurses and doctors who consulted her at the hospital? The whole process of caring for my loved one from one location to the next seemed so fragmented, and each caretaker seemed to have little concern or regard for my grandmother once she had left their walls. This entire process made very little sense to me. I was beyond baffled; I was angry.

It was what happened in the next few months that led to a significant change in my life. Just as I was growing frustrated with the lack of communication between my grandmother's caretakers several hundred miles away and while I was teaching night courses at a local university, one of my students approached me after class to ask if I would be interested in coming to work as the director of marketing and admissions for a skilled nursing facility in town. While it initially seemed like a huge leap, through much prayer and discussion with my wife, I decided to interview for the position. I was pleased to learn that the company, Life Care Centers of America, was a very reputable organization with facilities throughout the country. I also learned that they had an administrator-in-training (AIT) program designed to teach young professionals to be future health care leaders and operators.

Entering that nursing home for the first time proved to be a defining moment in my life and in my career. Still not convinced a switch to the nursing home industry was the change I had been waiting for, I entered the front doors of Life Care Center of Reno, Nevada, and there in the entry sat an elderly woman slouched over in a wheelchair. Not knowing if she needed assistance or not because she appeared to be unaware of her surroundings and slipping from her wheelchair, I stood in my tracks and pondered my next move. Should I help her? Is this normal for her? Is she in pain? Does she need assistance? While I did not know the answer to any of those questions, what became evident to me in that moment was that my reaction to this situation would no doubt shape and define who I would likely become as a health care leader.

God undoubtedly put this elderly woman in the entry that day to challenge me to stop and consider the task ahead. And while I did not know if the woman was in pain or needing assistance, it is what I did know in that moment that drove my decision to change my career. That day also laid the groundwork for how I would make decisions every day moving forward as a health care leader. My grandmother's misfortune led me to this place, and this woman was someone else's grandmother. I approached the woman, bent down to eye level with her, and with a smile asked if I could help her with anything. She said she was doing fine but thanked me for asking and smiled as I walked away. This was my first lesson in always remembering as a health care administrator that the patient's needs and care are always your top priority regardless of how busy you may think you are that day. Wearing your servant's heart on your sleeve at all times is nonnegotiable.

That moment in the entry and later walking into that nursing home for my first day of work were two of the most humbling experiences of my life. I would not trade those experiences for anything as they shaped me as a leader and, most importantly, gave me a personal confirmation of my own servant's heart. When I was ultimately offered the position, they agreed to accept me into a nationally recognized administrator-in-training program. And just like that, I made a career change and began learning the trade of becoming a health care administrator in a nursing home—a change that was inspired by my grandmother of all people. Just a few short years after marketing NBA players and PGA Tour professionals as well as flying on a private jet with one of the most recognizable sports figures in the world at the time, my focus had now turned to caring for compromised seniors who lived within the walls of a skilled nursing facility.

Later in my career, while serving as a hospital CEO and health system vice president, I often shared with my team members that it was the three weeks I spent washing dishes in the nursing home kitchen (during the dietary rotation of the nursing home training program) alongside individuals making minimum wage, which was less than six dollars an hour at the time, that taught me how to have respect for every employee who works in a health care facility.

Once the dietary training rotation was done, I completed a four-week rotation in the laundry department (once again with individuals making minimum wage) with some of the most content and happy employees I have ever worked alongside. My time in the laundry rotation helped me understand that there are more employees in a health care facility that can relate to the laundry and housekeeping staff than there are who can relate to someone in the administration like myself (with a college degree). I learned from those employees that they all shared one common characteristic: they all had a heart for caring and were proud to work at that facility because they knew they were making a difference in the lives of their patients. It was what I learned in that training program that taught me how to be a true health care leader.

Those early lessons as a young health care administrator showed me that the best way to lead a facility is to surround yourself with people who are subject-matter experts and empower them to do their job. I learned to treat all employees with respect and dignity, just as you or I would want to be treated. When conducting an interview to work in this environment, the one characteristic that each candidate must possess is to have a heart for caring. What is a heart for caring? It is having the passion for serving those in need, the elderly, or the physically challenged. When you meet a new job candidate, you can usually pick up on this characteristic within the first few seconds of the interview. This trait cannot be found on paper. In my mind, it is a nonnegotiable characteristic that all employees must possess. Oftentimes, this heart for caring becomes evident in a story about why they got into the field of health care. My story was my grandmother and the lack of focus on her as a patient that led to growing frustration within me. Most employees in the health care sector have a similar story that brought their servant's heart and empathy for those in need to the surface. Those are the candidates I sought out to identify as I ran health care facilities.

When someone has a heart for caring as most in the health care sector do, it shows in their smile, in their approach, in their demeanor, and in everything they do in every aspect of their life. This is why I am proud to be a health care administrator. It was my grandmother's resolve and heart for caring that God ultimately blessed me with as well, and I am thankful God led me to the health care sector as it is so rewarding to be an advocate for those most in need of health care services.

Less than three years into my health care career, I was asked to fill the role of chief executive officer (CEO) for a small, fledgling hospital in Southern California. While it is almost unheard of that a nursing home administrator would make the jump to manage an acute hospital, this hospital was a small hospital that simply tended to a few community members and a large number of nursing homes surrounding the property. The problem was that the nursing homes had lost confidence in this hospital's ability to properly care for patients in a quality manner and began telling ambulance drivers to drive right by the hospital and take their sick and emergent patients to a competing hospital. Thus, the ownership group thought a nursing home administrator like myself might have the skill set to turn their aging and fledgling hospital around.

Before being offered the job, I did some soul searching to give myself a clear sense of my motivation for having an interest in taking another path in my career. There was no doubt my salary potential could double, or even triple, if I made this move and established a career as an acute hospital CEO. Although that was tempting, I recognized that their aggressive approach to me was certainly flattering, and this showed their confidence in me. "But what about my residents?" I thought. "What about the very people I committed my career to when I left sports marketing a few years ago? What about the advocacy I had taken upon myself to get involved in—advocating for seniors, memory care support, and improved access to care?" I then took into consideration that the hospital I was considering to work for also had a small skilled nursing unit and a geriatric psychiatric unit. Before accepting the job, I asked to tour the nursing home unit and geropsychiatric unit, which were both off-site at a second campus.

As I toured the facility that day, being surrounded by aging seniors in a longer-term environment gave me confidence that my personal commitments and passion for serving this population were very much in need in this setting as well. The individual who offered me the job was also a former nursing home administrator, and we had some heartfelt discussions about my passion for serving the aging and those with memory impairment that I had grown to love in the SNF. Ultimately, they offered me the job, and I accepted. And within two years, the hospital was thriving.

Four years after I started in that role of CEO at Anaheim General Hospital, I was offered and accepted the same position at Western Medical Center Anaheim, a larger, competing hospital across town (now known as Anaheim Global Medical Center). In those roles, I would attend monthly gatherings of competing hospital executives and learn from their wisdom and experience. I did a lot of listening and very little talking. I knew I was learning on the job and wanted to earn the respect of my peers. From there, my career evolved to health-system-level positions and oversight of other post-acute levels of care including acute rehab, home health services, and hospice care. In short, my background is as well rounded as just about any health care professional you will meet. I am grateful for that fact and for the unique perspective it has given me.

In 2015, I was asked to teach at the University of Southern California's Sol Price School of Public Policy and in that same year became a best-selling health care author. My exciting journey is not over; it simply continues. Even after fifteen years in the health care industry, my sharing of my grandmother's story remains the same. The gifts of compassion and empathy that Grandma Belva passed on to me and the opportunity to lead, innovate, and collaborate with health care leaders across the country are gifts that I am thankful for, which have afforded me the platform to share these issues in this book with you, the reader.

After serving as an acute hospital chief executive officer, an acute rehab hospital chief executive officer, a health system vice president (overseeing hospice and home health), and a skilled nursing and assisted living facility administrator, I believe my experiences provide a thorough foundation to author this book. My experiences, combined with the expertise and knowledge of several trusted friends and colleagues from around the country who have contributed to this work, provide a thorough foundation for me to share perspectives on how to best meet your families' health care needs moving forward.

CHAPTER 2

The Fee-for-Service Free for All

According to Wikipedia (January 2016), fee-for-service (FFS) is a payment model where services are unbundled and paid for separately. In health care, it gives an incentive for physicians to provide more treatments because quality is dependent on the quantity of care rather than the quality of care. Similarly, when patients are shielded from paying (cost-sharing) by health insurance coverage, they are incentivized to welcome any medical service that might do some good. FFS is the dominant physician payment method in the United States. It raises costs and discourages the efficiencies of integrated care, and a variety of reform efforts have been attempted, recommended, or initiated to reduce its influence.

HAVE YOU EVER heard anyone say, "I can't wait to be admitted to a nursing home someday"? Most people chuckle when I make that statement. And that's fair. It's a laughable statement. Of course, no human being wants to be admitted to a skilled nursing facility. You could likely say the same for an acute hospital. It would be unlikely to hear someone state that they look forward to their next injury or accident so they can visit the emergency room or acute hospital. Perhaps some of our aging physicians should be reminded of this.

Medicare is the federal insurance program for Americans over the age of sixty-five. In recent years, approximately 22 percent of all Medicare patients admitted to an acute hospital are subsequently transferred to an institutionalized level of post-acute care (nursing home, long-term acute care hospital, or acute rehab hospital). Although on the surface one would assume a doctor would only send a patient from the hospital to another institution as a last resort, that is not always the case (as a result of financial incentives). Thus, one reason for such a high volume of patients being transferred from hospitals to post-acute institutions instead of being discharged home is that their doctor is incentivized financially to keep them institutionalized. To further explain, the origins of the fee-for-service reimbursement model in America are discussed below and date back to the pre-World War II era.

Perhaps Dr. Atul Gawande's story of negotiating his first salary as a Harvard surgeon best describes the fee-for-service model. Gawande became well known among health care executives and physicians in 2014 when his book *Being Mortal* was published. Gawande describes eighteenth century BC Babylon where surgeons received ten shekels for lifesaving operations on citizens and two shekels for the same operation on slaves.

Dr. Gawande also penned a *New Yorker* article about the results of the fee-for-service delivery model in McAllen, Texas, where one doctor stated, "Medicine has become a pig trough here. We took a wrong turn when doctors stopped being doctors and became businessmen."[1] Gawande's article provides a great description of the fee-for-service approach and the standardized fee schedule that was created in the 1980s to pay doctors for each of the different services they provide both in hospitals and in their offices. This is the same manner in which hospitals billed for services in the fee-for-service era.

I think it is fair to state a few facts here. First, I share many similar beliefs and approaches with Dr. Gawande. Second, it is only fair to point out that the majority of doctors practicing today have been conditioned to this model and accompanying behavior. In fact, with the exception of the most experienced physicians who are nearing retirement, many Generation X doctors have never known any other method beyond fee-for-service. With that in mind, it is imperative that

---

[1] http://www.newyorker.com/archive/2005/04/04/050404fa_fact

doctors understand the goals of health care reform and advocate for financial models that allow them to continue to provide the necessary care and also generate a justifiable income.

There are a number of problems with the fee-for-service approach. The methodology, as described above, undoubtedly incentivizes and results in overutilization of services and delivery of expensive, unnecessary care. The fee-for-service model financially incentivizes doctors to admit patients to hospitals and post-acute facilities and further rewards them financially for keeping patients in facilities for extended lengths of time. Not to mention, primary-care doctors take care of their buddies or fellow physicians by referring often unnecessary tests to them as specialists, which allows these specialists to bill for services as well. While this is not the case for all physicians of course, it is widely accepted and understood that this takes place in hospitals with a significant number of independent physicians who are not affiliated with or compensated by a larger group but rely strictly on widgets, *errrr* (yes, I made this sound up), the volume of patients seen daily, for their income.

Think about it. Let's provide a hypothetical example of a sixty-five-year-old male. The man calls his longtime family doctor, and this is what takes place:

> Patient calls doctor: "Hey, Doc, I fell a week ago, and my hip is still hurting. Should I come see you or go straight to an orthopedic specialist?"

> Family doctor responds: "Come see me first. I will let you know if you need to see a specialist." (This is the first unnecessary step in the process, but now the primary-care physician gets to bill the payer.)

> Patient visits family doctor at his office: Family doctor examines patient and refers patient to the hospital for labs and imaging tests. Family doctor bills payer ($) for office visit.

Patient goes to hospital for labs and imaging tests: Hospital bills payer for services provided ($).

Hospital calls family doctor with results: The doctor's fishing expedition (to find any issue with the patient he can) pays off as he finds some minor swelling and a possible minor hairline fracture in one image.

Family doctor refers patient to orthopedic specialist: Orthopedic specialist says he only has office hours two days a week, so it's best to meet him at the hospital. Advises patient to go back to the hospital but to report to the emergency room and advise the nurse that the orthopedic specialist told him to come to the emergency department.

Patient goes to emergency department: Patient reports to the nurse his minor hip discomfort from a week-old injury and that the orthopedic specialist advised him to go to the emergency department. Nurse calls orthopedic specialist, who orders additional x-rays and an MRI but does not have time to come to the hospital until twelve hours later as he has other priorities. Hospital bills for emergency services, MRI, and x-ray ($).

Nurse calls orthopedic specialist: Nurse advises orthopedic specialist that the images have been returned. Radiology doctor hired by the hospital documents that there is a possible hairline fracture but is unsure. Radiologist bills payer for reading images ($).

Patient admitted to the hospital: Orthopedic specialist orders the patient admitted to the hospital for observation and requests that the family doctor or assigned hospital primary-care doctor perform the initial required history and physical upon admission.

Hospital doctor (hospitalist) does history and physical on patient as the family doctor was unavailable to drive over to the hospital that night. Hospitalist is unable to find any pertinent information about the patient documented in the notes or chart, so he/she asks the emergency department nurse why the patient is there, and she reports, "He fell a week ago and has minor pain in his hip. There may be a hairline fracture. The orthopedic specialist thinks the patient may need hip surgery and wants to evaluate him as a precaution." The hospitalist, who thinks a different exam may be more effective than those images already taken, orders an additional image done and notices some lab results slightly out of range. The hospitalist then orders a consult by a cardiologist. The hospitalist bills the payer ($).

Orthopedic specialist finally arrives at the hospital: Orthopedic specialist examines the patient, who has been at the hospital for ten hours now, and does not see any need to keep the patient hospitalized any longer. He advises the patient to take Motrin but wants to hold off on discharging the patient until the cardiologist completes his consult. Orthopedic specialist bills the payer ($).

Cardiologist completes consult: Cardiologist consults patient, finds no reason for concern, and discharges the patient home after twelve hours in the hospital. The cardiologist ($) and the hospital ($) bill for services.

All because the patient had a sore hip and needed Motrin. Do you wonder now why the Medicare fund is running dry and insurers require preauthorization for services? What if the patient had simply gone to the orthopedic specialist's office first? The result would have been identical as each of those tests was unnecessary. This practice still continues today.

The key operational flaw in the fee-for-service delivery model is that there is no required preauthorization for services. The term "managed care" emerged in the 1980s as a means to control this type of *laissez-faire* behavior by requiring the insurer to preauthorize any services ordered by a doctor or hospital. Without preauthorization, the doctor and provider do not get paid. There are many forms of managed care, but the one constant that is a cost control measure is a written preauthorization from the insurer.

Without a required preauthorization, the delivery model was lawless, and much abuse took place. Fraud ran rampant in the health care sector as greedy owners and physicians took advantage of an environment with no one at the helm. Thus, I have personally renamed the fee-for-service era **"the fee-for-service free for all!"**

In an era with explosive growth in the health care space where there could not possibly have beenenough oversight, the fee-for-service era truly became a free-for-all, and it was lucrative for many. The problem was that the federal Medicare fund was disappearing at an alarming, unsustainable rate, and there was little evidence justifying that this increase in spending was resulting in improved health or improved quality. Read on.

CHAPTER 3

The Post-Acute Merry-Go-Round

L ET ME START this chapter by saying that the practices I am describing in these early chapters are not necessarily the norm for all practicing physicians. I am providing examples that will help illustrate the ill-willed incentives of the fee-for-service model. Let me point out that most doctors taking the time to read this book are likely not doctors who employ these practices as those who consciously or unconsciously operate in financially motivated manners are usually not the same individuals spending their leisure time reading to sharpen their sword and hone their craft. In fact, they likely use their free time to identify other means of financially maximizing opportunities rather than how to best stay true to their Hippocratic oath. So in short, this book is by no means an attempt to state that certain types of physician behavior are true for all doctors but simply that those who are exploiting the system essentially ruined it for everyone.

Doctors who are employed or are part of a medical group have less incentive to operate in this manner as they receive a salary in many cases. There are, however, quite a few doctors who prefer to remain independent so that they can practice as individual business owners. As a result, independent practice doctors have much more incentive to bill as many patients as possible and order as many tests as possible.

To be fair, it was not just doctors that were incentivized to institutionalize. Hospitals and post-acute facilities shared the same incentive. The fee-for-service era was also the "heads-in-beds" era. That is how providers were reimbursed. The Affordable Care Act (ACA) was designed in large part to end the heads-in-beds mentality and disincentivize unnecessary hospitalization and unnecessary institutionalization in post-acute facilities. Essentially, almost every care coordination incentive and penalty in the ACA was implemented to prevent unnecessary hospitalization and institutionalization. In short, the federal government states, "If you admit someone to a hospital or nursing home that did not need to be there and could have been cared for at a lower level of care, we are not going to pay you, and we are also going to fine you."

This is not just true for institutions, but it is also true for Medicare-reimbursed home health services. The government clearly states, "If the patient does not need the services, we will not be reimbursing you for them." In fact, although home health services are the lowest cost level of care and at the heart of the delivery model of the future, there has been rampant fraud in the home health sector, and the federal government watches this sector closely.

In the fee-for-service era, doctors learned quickly that the financial fruits of overadmitting and overutilizing (extending patient's length of stay in facilities) were plentiful. This led to what has turned into a broken system. Even more fruitful than the doctor's income was that of the owner of skilled nursing, acute rehab, and long-term acute care hospitals as thousands of facilities sprung up across the country. Each time criteria or methodology changed, physicians and owners would study the changes and adapt.

It was "the fee-for-service free for all," and it was lucrative for all. The reality is that in a capitalistic society, those who are first to market often see significant financial rewards. The intent of this book is not to place blame but to break down the new model, the post-ACA model. The post-ACA model is completely contrary to the fee-for-service model, and those who are first to adapt to a value-based model will reap the financial benefit.

Similar to the unnecessary hospitalization described in the prior chapter, let's look at the incentives for providers and doctors when a patient, particularly a senior, is admitted to the hospital. Let's use my late grandmother Belva's story from the last summer of her life as an example.

In the summer of 2001, my late grandmother's congestive heart failure was progressing, so she ended up in the hospital. As discussed earlier, both the doctor and the provider (the hospital in this case) got paid for her care during the stay. Rather than ask her if she felt strong enough to go home as home-based support services were available, the doctor placed his own personal financial interests ahead of my grandmother's preferences and advised her that she needed to be "transferred to" what is known as a long-term acute care hospital (LTACH) to continue her recovery. Doctors are very skilled at using terms like "transfer" instead of "discharge" as "discharge" may suggest the patient has a choice in the matter. The truth is, the patient always has a choice in the matter. But for some reason in America, patients are either not aware of that fact or are afraid to speak up.

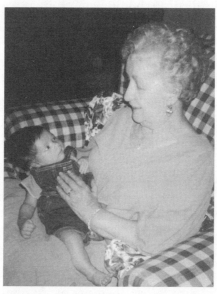

My grandma Belva Riddle holds her newborn great-grandson shortly before she entered the hospital in 2001.

So when my grandmother arrived at the LTACH, she was surprised to learn that she would be staying for more than three weeks. Needless to say, she was disappointed. As was I—she appeared to me to be healthy enough to go home. But remember, both the doctor and the provider get paid at this stop too. In fact, the doctor often gets paid an additional monthly stipend ranging from $1,000 to $4,000 a month to provide "services" to the LTACH that its operators deem important and necessary. Many of these services have been legally challenged as unnecessary. But more importantly, the monthly stipend is seen as a means to incentivize and motivate hospital doctors to refer patients to post-acute facilities such as LTACH. The "wink-and-the-nod" between the post-acute provider and the doctor is that these monthly stipends are paid, and in return, the doctor refers as many patients as possible so that the beds remain full. This clearly clouds the doctor's ability to provide unbiased input to patients in the hospital as there is significant pressure to keep post-acute beds full.

After three weeks and four days in the long-term acute care, my grandmother was then advised that she needed to continue her care in a "rehab facility." It should be no surprise to anyone that my grandmother stayed exactly twenty-five days, as twenty-five days is the average length of stay required to maximize Medicare reimbursement and maintain licensure for LTACHs. The bigger providers got so good at managing this length of stay within an average range of twenty-four to twenty-six days that the *Wall Street Journal* documented the egregiousness of this financially driven practice which could not be linked to any sort of quality improvement.[2]

So after four weeks away from home in two different hospital settings, my grandmother reacted to the news of another "transfer" by stating, "I thought I was rehabbing here. What is a rehab facility?" The reality is it's a fancy name for a convalescent home or a nursing home. In fact, the long-term care industry has gone to great lengths in recent years to shed both of those names, replacing them with the name skilled nursing facility and short-term rehab facility. Why? There are two reasons for that.

1) Nursing home reimbursement for short-term therapy days is two to four times ($300–$700) greater per day than the reimbursement operators receive for long-term custodial patients ($150–$200).

---

2   By Christopher Weaver, Anna Wilde Mathews and Tom McGinty: Feb. 17, 2015; http://www.wsj.com/articles/hospital-discharges-rise-at-lucrative-times-1424230201

2) As stated earlier, no one wants to go to a convalescent home or nursing home, so let's change the semantics, and perhaps patients in the hospital and their family members will not understand where we are sending their loved one until they actually get to the nursing home.

Without straying too far from the point being made here, once she arrived at the convalescent home, *errrr* (yes, there's that made-up sound again!), I mean, skilled nursing facility (SNF), once again, both the doctor and the provider (SNF) get paid at this stop as well. Now you might be asking, how long does this go on before Grandma Belva gets to go home? Great question. The answer to that question should be the same whether she is in a hospital, doctor's office, LTACH, or SNF. The question is, "Is Grandma Belva able to return home safely, and if so, what resources might she require in the home to ensure she will be safe to recover and rehabilitate?" During the fee-for-service era, doctors rarely asked that question as it would have been financially prohibitive. In fact, each time my grandmother got passed to a different level of care, the financial incentives changed and in a sense started all over again for both the new provider and the doctor.

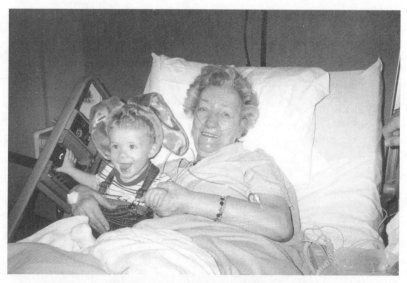

Grandma Belva again with my oldest son from her bed in a long-term acute care hospital. The next day, she penned the letter on the following page.

Dear Martine and Josh and Branton 8-16-01

You have no idea how much it meant to me to have you all come by last night. I am sure the Lord will bless you for taking your precious time to do it.

I am so proud of all three of you - and happy to know how the Spirit of God dwells in your home. You have truly been blessed with such a gorgeous child. He is just beautiful - and his penetrating smile. I can't believe how big he is. He's a little boy - not a baby. I'm sure his baby brother will be just like he is. That shows you what Love can do.

Today it is very hot here and I'm thinking of you at the beach enjoying yourself. I am sure you are having a wonderful time.

I'm getting anxious now to get home and get settled. Four months is a long time to be away from home. The longest in my whole life.

Thank you again for coming and taking me out to dinner. It was a great evening.

Love to all
Grandma

XOXOXOXOXO XO XO XOXOXO XOXOXOXO

My grandmother wrote this letter to me from the hospital after being institutionalized in different facilities for four months. Note the second-to-last paragraph (with the two lines and arrow at the left that illustrates her making this comment).

So once Grandma Belva was transferred to a skilled nursing facility frankly because she was led by her physician to feel that she did not have a choice in the matter, the very sweet social worker at the skilled nursing facility advised her that they were hopeful she could heal fast enough to return home after three weeks. Three weeks! Why three weeks? Well, you are getting keen on how the system worked at this point. There are two reasons SNF providers strive for a twenty-day length of stay:

1. SNFs are reimbursed in seven-day episodes based on the minutes of therapy provided in those seven days. After the seventh day, the patient's rehab minutes are totaled, and a per diem is decided for those days. If the episode is cut shorter than five days and the patient is discharged home, it becomes difficult for SNFs to achieve the desired weekly therapy minutes and corresponding lucrative reimbursement.

2. After twenty days, patients are required to start paying a daily co-pay, and miraculously, once advised of this, most patients insist on returning home that day. Once again, with little evidence to show a quality link to twenty-day stays, most SNFs have an average length of stay just under twenty days for rehab patients.

The longer a patient stays and participates in therapy, the more reimbursement the SNF receives at the lucrative rehab rates. Most patients plateau and no longer show rehab improvement between the tenth and seventeenth day in an SNF. Thus, SNFs try to maximize reimbursement by pacing the patient at a twenty-day rate to lengthen the projected stay and maximize the SNF's reimbursement.

Providers' Desired Length of Stay (LOS) in Each Level of Care to Maximize Financial Opportunity

Hospital →	LTACH →	Acute Rehab →	Skilled Nursing →	Home Health →	Independent at Home
3–5 days (Varies)	(25 days)	10–14 days (varies)	20 days fully paid for by Medicare: Up to 100 days covered in total	Most episodes are 6 to 8 weeks (3 days a week for an hour on average)	* This is the desired outcome for all levels of care listed.

LOS = length of stay

And let us not forget the two financial incentives for physicians to refer patients to the skilled nursing facility. They are identical to the two incentives in LTACH:

1. Not only does the doctor get paid again for consulting the patient in a new facility (SNF),
2. but the doctor often collects a monthly per diem ($1,000–$4,000) from the skilled nursing facility as well.

Again, this monthly stipend is often a sham, a handshake agreement that is allegedly in place for the doctor to perform "needed services" for the SNF, when in actuality, the understanding is that the doctor will refer a high volume of patients and keep the SNF's beds full. Needless to say, at the SNF level, just as other levels of care, both the doctor and the provider bill for services.

Finally, after three weeks in the SNF, my grandmother was miraculously finally ready to return home. However, the doctor advised her that unless she was willing to participate in home health therapy services, she would have to reside in the nursing home for the rest of her life. Wow! What a way to package two options for a senior to choose from. Door number 1 please! "I will go home with home health services," she said. And yes, you guessed it, not only does the doctor get a monthly stipend from the home health agency (to refer patients of course), but the provider and the physician once again bill the insurer.

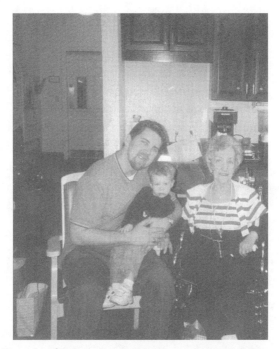

Grandma Belva pictured here at an assisted living facility with Josh Luke and his oldest son.

It's the fee-for-service free for all, no doubt about it. And guess what happened a month later when my grandmother fell and was rushed to the emergency department? Well, if you were listening very carefully, back in Southern California in the summer of 2001, you may have heard a collective cheer from the provider and physician community when my grandmother arrived back at the emergency room. Yep, it was time to put her back on the forty-five-day merry-go-round again and let all providers and doctors bill for delivering services to her. Imagine a world where providers and physicians actually just met her basic needs and comforted her emotionally so she could return home safely to age and heal in her own environment. The illustration titled "Grandma Belva, Congestive Heart Failure, Summer of 2002" illustrates this service-driven model.

The irony of this summer, and the accompanying graphic, is that she did not live long enough to be put on hospice services once she returned to the hospital. The reality was that was easily the next step in the process of her care. And yes, you guessed it, the incentives for both the provider and the physician were identical. Providers and physicians don't get paid when you are healthy, so patients are often institutionalized unnecessarily for financial gain—whether willfully or not. It is very likely that home-based services could have been offered and could have improved her care while at the same time saving significant Medicare dollars. Guess what else? My grandmother would have been much happier being cared for in her home than at those different facilities. The problem? No one ever advised her that home-based care was an option. Why would they—it was not in their best interest.

Read on.

Grandma Belva—Congestive Heart Failure

The Summer of 2002

Medicare dollars paid to providers. Does not include doctor!

Home	$0
Hospital	$48,000
LTACH	$52,000
Nursing Home	$12,000
Home with Home Health	$4,000
Hospital	$36,000
Nursing Home	$18,000
Assisted Living with Home Health	$4,000
Hospital	$42,000
Nursing Home	$24,000
Hospital	$58,000
Total Costs of Care	**$298,000**

CHAPTER 4

The Quota-Based Physician:
Forget about Your Health,
It's about Your Doctor's Income

A GAIN LET ME start this chapter with a clarification: what I am about to share with you is more so pointing a finger at specialty post-acute hospital owners and operators, not at physicians. Physicians are almost like guinea pigs in the specialty hospital incentivization experiment—guinea pigs that "shifted to the dark side" in a model that proved to be extremely lucrative for all. And these guinea pigs shared in the financial windfall of the model just as much as the specialty hospital owners and CEOs who were pulling in $3-$11 million annual compensation packages at times. And one last point, while not illegal in practice, at the very minimum, what is described in this chapter is not patient-centric and borders on unethical. The reality is that this "quota-based physician-ing" practice became so entrenched in some doctors' daily routine that it became the norm, and they would hesitate to even suggest it is true. Plausible deniability perhaps?

Now that you have read the prior chapter, "The Post-acute Merry-go-round," you have a basic understanding for physician and provider financial incentives. With that in mind, would you believe the most egregious incentive to put the doctor's interest above that of the patient's has not yet been revealed? So what is quota-based physician-ing? Read on.

Doctors are legally able to bill Medicare and other insurers daily for care delivered in a long-term acute care hospital (LTACH) or an inpatient rehab facility (IRF). However, in a skilled nursing facility, since it is deemed a lower level of care and not "acute" like the others, doctors are only allowed to bill Medicare once a month after the initial "history and physical" is completed upon admission to the SNF. Additionally, in-home health doctors are permitted to bill even less than once a month.

Thus, the more patients a doctor transfers from the acute hospital to an LTACH or IRF, the more personal income a physician can earn. While it is rare and not a widely accepted approach, I have nicknamed this type of patient management by physicians "quota-based physician-ing." It was prevalent during the fee-for-service era and led to significant wasteful spending of Medicare dollars.

So instead of considering sending the patient home as an option for discharge when a patient is hospitalized, active doctors who focused on caring for senior citizens became entrenched in a culture that is more based on what they argued "limited physician liability" by erring on the side of caution and sending patients to institutions after the hospital instead of to their homes. "I cannot send this patient home as it is my liability on the line if they fall and get hurt once they get home," a doctor might say. Those are pretty powerful words. They are certainly words that are slow to be challenged by any nonphysician. The word "liability" usually ends the conversation as no one would challenge the physician. It is the same word emergency room doctors use to justify admitting patients to the hospital as opposed to discharging them home from the emergency department. Another example of wasted Medicare dollars in the fee-for-service era.

The financial incentive for doctors to practice quota-based physician-ing is significant. Doctors are taught these financially lucrative tactics by the very specialty hospitals that they refer patients to. These specialty hospitals, long-term acute care hospitals, and acute rehab hospitals pay them a monthly stipend for providing allegedly "necessary" physician quality and support services. To further this point, when one of these services contracts expires (usually annually), if the doctor had not been referring a significant volume of patients to the LTACH or IRF, their services agreement will not likely be renewed. Guess what? Once those "services" are no longer performed, there is no noticeable impact on the facility, its operations, its quality, or its patient satisfaction. So I ask you, if the services are "needed" to justify them legally, why is it that when they are no longer performed, no one misses a beat? It is all a sham, that's why.

Acute hospitals use this same "directorship" for the needed services approach to ensure doctors choose their hospital over others when referring patients from the hospital to their private practice. Look no further than Tri-City Regional Hospital in Oceanside, California, which received a healthy fine from the federal government for this very issue in late 2015.

How lucrative are the financial rewards of employing a quota-based approach for an independently practicing physician? Let's take a look at the following illustration. The graph shows that an active doctor who averages a census of ten patients a day in acute hospitals and will send most home upon discharge unless they absolutely need to rehabilitate at an SNF would receive reimbursement from Medicare of just under $279,000 annually. However, if that same doctor instituted a quota-based approach and found a justification to transfer as many of those patients as possible to an LTACH, he would receive approximately $672,000 annually in Medicare reimbursement. It is more than double the income. Sounds like a perfect material for a future episode of *American Greed*!

Quota-based physicians are also notorious for having an acute hospital length of stay that is longer than the norm. The reason they do this is, as always, financially motivated. Even though the patient may be healthy enough to go home after being in the hospital for three days, the physician is often able to collect one to two more days of reimbursement if the patient stays in the hospital. As awful as it sounds, your doctor could leave you in a hospital unnecessarily so he or she can collect an additional $55 in reimbursement. Welcome to the American health care delivery model that is fee-for-service.

The Quota-Based Physician:
This Chart provides an Example of a Doctor Who Attempts to Transfer All Patients from the Acute Hospital To a Long Term Acute Care Hospital (LTACH) or Acute Rehab
(Physicians Annual Income: app. $672,100)

	Acute Hospital	LTACH or IRF	SNF	Total Patient Consults Per Day
New Admits (higher reimbursement on day 1 of admit)	$140 Per Patient on first day for History & Physical 3 new admits a day = $420 a day Weekly reimbursement ($420 x 7) = $2,940	$140 Per Patient on first day for History & Physical 3 new admits a day = $420 a day (transferred from hospital) Weekly reimbursement ($420 x 7) = $2,940	$140 Per Patient on first day for History & Physical Total weekly H & P: 2 Weekly reimbursement ($140 x 2) = $280	Total Weekly H & P: 44 Weekly reimbursement = $6,160
Census	$55 per consult 7 Patient Consults a Day = $385 a day Weekly reimbursement ($385 x 7) = $2,695	$55 per consult 10 Patient Consults a Day = $550 a day Weekly reimbursement ($550 x 7) = $3,850	$55 per consult Weekly Consults (4): $220 Weekly reimbursement ($55 x 4) = $220	Total Weekly Consults: 123 Weekly reimbursement = $6,765
Total Daily Reimbursement	Daily Acute Hospital Reimbursement = $805 Weekly reimbursement ($805 x 7) = $5,635	Daily LTACH/IRF Reimbursement = $970 Weekly reimbursement ($970 x 7) = $6,790	Weekly Combined SNF Reimbursement = $500	Total Combined Weekly Reimbursement = $12,925
Total Annual Reimbursement	Annual hospital reimbursement = $293,020	Annual LTACH/IRF reimbursement = $353,080	Total annual reimbursement $26,000	**Total annual reimbursement $672,100**

Based on the same daily acute hospital census (left column) as the chart on the opposite page, the Quota-based physician earns approximately $672,000 a year in Medicare reimbursement, even though many of the patients that were transferred to LTACH or IRF could have likely been transferred directly home from the hospital or to a nursing home for a few days.

The Non-Quota-Based Physician:
This Chart provides an Example of a Doctor Who Attempts to "Do the Right Thing" & get Patients Transferred Home from the hospital when possible
(Physicians Annual Income: app. $278,980)

	Acute Hospital	LTACH or IRF	SNF	Total Patient Consults Per Day
New Admits (higher reimbursement on day 1 of admit)	140 Per Patient on first day for History & Physical 3 new admits a day = $420 a day Weekly reimbursement ($420 x 7) = $2,940	0 new admits a day (transferred from hospital) Weekly reimbursement = $0	$140 Per Patient on first day for History & Physical Total weekly H & P: 2 Weekly reimbursement ($140 x 2) = $280	Total Weekly H & P: 23 Weekly reimbursement = $3,220
Census	$55 per consult 5 Patient Consults a Day = $385 a day Weekly reimbursement ($385 x 5) = $1,925	0 Consults a Day = $0 a day Weekly reimbursement = $0	$55 per consult Weekly Consults (4): $220 Weekly reimbursement ($55 x 4) = $220	Total Weekly Consults: 39 Weekly reimbursement = $2,145
Total Daily Reimbursement	Daily Acute Hospital Reimbursement = $805 Weekly reimbursement ($805 x 7) = $4,865	Daily LTACH/IRF Reimbursement = $0 Weekly reimbursement = $0	Weekly Combined SNF Reimbursement = $500	Total Combined Weekly Reimbursement = $5,365
Total Annual Reimbursement	Annual Hospital Reimbursement = $252,980	Annual LTACH/IRF Reimbursement = 0	Annual SNF Reimbursement $26,000	**Total Annual Reimbursement $278,980**

Based on the same daily acute hospital (left column) census as the chart on the opposite page, the non-Quota-based physician earns approximately $278,980 a year in Medicare reimbursement, as his or her goal is to attempt to transfer patients directly home from the acute hospital, or in a worst case transfer them to a nursing home for a few days before going home.

I operated and consulted for several hospitals in which case managers and discharge planners reported examples of this taking place regularly. It is downright awful. Even worse is that cash-strapped hospitals serving the inner city are often helpless to change the doctor's behavior even when they have egregious examples. These hospitals are so desperate to put heads in beds so they can bill that they are not about to bite the hand that feeds them by alienating a high-volume-referring physician. It would be career suicide for any hospital CEO to do so. Even though it's an almost inhumane practice, the hospital is helpless in many cases to address it.

Can you imagine finishing medical school and residency then looking across the table at your spouse, partner, or parent to discuss future plans and not being intrigued by the quota-based approach? Imagine this statement from a soon-to-be doctor to his or her loved one: I can follow my dream and practice medicine in the office and at the hospital and pull in just under $279,000 annually, or I could institute this model that this specialty hospital (LTACH or IRF) organization just showed me and make $672,000 annually instead by seeing patients in the hospital and post-acute facilities.

Can you imagine? Student loans and years of mounting debt to pay off and an individual is faced with this decision. For many young doctors, they may not realize it at the time, but that decision may be the most important career decision they ever made. Its impact will infiltrate all aspects of the doctor's future practice, care delivery, business decision, and household income. It is a moment of truth. A true life-changing decision. So what do you think is the result for the doctor who chooses to remain independent? It is quota-based physician-ing of course, and you can thank the large specialty hospitals for educating young physicians about this lucrative opportunity. I know. I worked for several of the large specialty hospitals and was trained to train doctors on these financial opportunities!

As it relates to documentation, physicians can essentially justify anything they desire as long as they have a game plan from the start. Physicians know which tests to order to create a logical path to suggesting someone needs a LTACH visit after the hospital. Even in the absence of any outcome justification, the mere fact that physicians are considered experts, as well as their ability to document "toward" the discharge instead of documenting the true facts, is enough reason for everyone to look the other way in the fee-for-service era. I call this "documenting toward your desired disposition." It runs rampant in hospitals and post-acute facilities where nurses and administrators often feel helpless to question a doctor's judgement and is a means for a doctor to paint a picture that suggests post-acute care is needed by simply knowing which words to write in a chart.

One of the questions this book aims to answer is simple: "Are we able to transform our delivery model to a truly patient-centered delivery model?" If yes, the first question to be asked by doctors when patients are hospitalized should simply be this: "Can this patient be cared for at home, and if so, what resources are needed to ensure a safe discharge?" Remember this when you or a loved one goes to the hospital: You have a choice every step of the way. Feel empowered to question the doctor when something is not completely clear.

The biggest challenge during the fee-for-service era, as alluded to the story of my grandmother, was that no one ever educated her or the family that she had a choice in where to go after her hospital stay. They also never asked her if she wanted to go at all or if she preferred to go home.

If you take away just a few nuggets from this book, let one of them be this: This is America, and as patients, whether in the fee-for-service era or in post-ACA, you ultimately have a choice in who will be your provider and what type of care you will be given. God bless, America!

CHAPTER 5

What Ever Happened to the Personal Family Physician?

REMEMBER THE DAYS of having a personal family physician? You could call him or her in the middle of the night and walk into their office anytime without an appointment, and they would meet you at the hospital when you were injured or ill. Well, those days are rapidly coming to an end.

The age of physician specialization is upon us. Most family doctors and primary-care physicians are no longer credentialed to even care for patients in a hospital setting, let alone a post-acute setting. The financial structure and incentives of the fee-for-service era led doctors to choose their preferred business model. Very few still have an active office practice and care for patients in the hospital. In fact, the few doctors who maintain an active office practice and also see patients in hospitals and post-acute facilities almost entirely have hired partners, nurse practitioners, or physicians assistants to support them in adequately fulfilling all these obligations.

So while you may still have a personal family physician, it is likely that your physician would not care for you should you be admitted to the hospital. So who then cares for you in the hospital? A hospitalist.

Medicare began reimbursing hospitals on an episode-based methodology during the fee-for-service era. This means that regardless of how long the patient remained in the hospital, the hospital was being paid a flat rate depending on the patient's severity and comorbidities.

Thus, hospitals quickly realized that the shorter length of time that a patient was in the hospital, the more profitable the hospital would be for that patient's care. Managing a patient's "length of stay" became a top priority. Many primary-care physicians, who in the 1990s were still caring for their patients when they were hospitalized, had a tough time meeting the hospitals' demand to shorten length of stay.

For example, hospital nursing and physician teams conduct rounds each morning and review each patient in the hospital. If during morning rounds the care team determines that a patient is ready to be discharged or will be ready by the day's end, the physician is notified as he or she is required to write a discharge order in the chart before the patient is eligible for discharge. For private-practice doctors, if the hospitals calls at 10:00 a.m. to advise a patient is ready and needs a discharge order written, the doctor may not be able to get to the hospital until that night to write the order. This is known as a discharge delay. In some cases, the doctor was not planning to visit the hospital at all that day and would wait until the next morning.

Hospitals quickly realized that they could not rely on these private-practice physicians to reply and write discharge orders in a timely manner. Thus, hospitals began contracting for "hospitalist" services. A hospitalist is a doctor who is contracted with the hospital for the sole purpose of managing patients in that hospital. One of their main goals and their top priority each day is to identify patients who are ready for discharge and make sure the patients are discharged in a timely manner.

Over time, this practice became more and more common to the point that many hospitals converted to an entirely hospitalist model and no longer permitted private-practice physicians to consult patients within the hospital. The hospitalist model is even more prevalent in a managed care environment, so it is likely to continue being the norm in a post-ACA environment. In fact, most managed care organizations do not use the hospital's hospitalist group but contract with their own group of doctors, or "hospitalists," to ensure that doctors have aligned incentives with the managed care organization and not the hospital.

So that's the reason why you can't see your personal family physician when you go to the hospital. He or she is no longer credentialed to care for you in the hospital!

To take that point even further, physician specialization has evolved as post-acute doctors have employed a hospitalist model as well. These contracted post-acute specialists are referred to as "SNFists." In most cases, these contracted SNFists do not have a private practice and do not care for patients in hospitals. They simply spend their entire day consulting patients in SNFs and other post-acute facilities.

It is ironic when you think about it. Hospitals are contracted with hospitalist groups in the fee-for-service era for two very specific reasons:

1) First and foremost, admit as many patients as possible to drive as much inpatient revenue as possible to the hospital.
2) Once a patient is admitted to the hospital, immediately start planning and developing a care plan to discharge the patient as soon as possible.

That's it. That was the secret to running a hospital in the fee-for-service era! Another way to look at it would be to say that the role of the hospitalist in the fee-for-service era was simply to "Get 'em in and then get 'em out!"

And this is why the days of a personal family physician who cares for all levels of need have gone by the wayside.

CHAPTER 6

The ACA Marks the End of the Golden Age of Hospital Profitability

CORRECT ME IF I am wrong, but weren't we led to believe that one of the many reasons America needed health care reform was to lessen the influence of insurance companies? Inflating profits and profit margins in the 1990s and 2000s spiraled out of control as managed care organizations became more and more efficient. So seven years after the passing of the Affordable Care Act (ACA), do you think it has lessened the influence and profit margins of insurers? That's a laugher! While physicians started selling their independent practices and joining larger medical groups prior to 2010, the ratification of the ACA all but wiped out any influence physicians had in the delivery model, with hospitals and health systems not far behind.

After the passing of the ACA, health care executives quickly realized that the hospital was no longer the center point of the health care delivery system. The post-ACA model focuses on the three aims of health care: (1) a healthier population, (2) improved medical care, and (3) reduced costs and efficiencies in delivering care. It was only a matter of a few months before reputable hospitals started discussing how to more aggressively pursue this model. One of the first trends that emerged was hospitals purchasing medical groups. Why, you ask? That's a good question. With such a drastic change forthcoming, hospitals and health systems had more access to capital than most medical groups. Thus, the race began between hospitals and doctors to see who could claim the power position in the unexplored new model. Health systems also assumed that taking ownership of physician practices would eliminate one potential challenger in the struggle for power as physicians have become increasingly adept at finding ways to compete with hospitals in recent years. Furthermore, health systems purchasing physician practices was at a minimum a defensive strategy in securing market share from competitors. As a result of some of the recommended new payment models in the ACA, physicians would gain leverage over health systems with regard to which hospital they might choose to send patients, so many health systems just chose to eliminate that possibility as a risk factor and acquired physician groups.

In addition, another trend that emerged shortly after the ACA passed was that a number of successful and deep-rooted community hospitals announced plans to close acute hospitals and to convert campuses into outpatient settings. Other health systems kept hospitals open, but they restructured them to provide new outpatient and ambulatory services that had traditionally been provided in the inpatient setting. This was all done with the goal in mind of allowing a wider variety of outpatient services that would better allow patients to age and heal at home.

As a result of these trends and the incentives in the ACA, hospitals started to realize that without being part of a system or a network, the hospital business was going to change dramatically. That change did not appear to be a favorable one financially as the incentives in the ACA reward organizations that keep people well and out of the hospital. Thus, without other service lines that generate revenue that can contribute to the bottom line, the delivery model of the future will make it extremely difficult for stand-alone providers or individual hospitals.

Between 2012 and 2015, this became more evident to stand-alone hospitals as the impact of the added penalties started to take their toll on these types of providers. This trend led to a series of mergers and acquisitions and, in some cases, closure. In short, the model of the future requires a wide array of services to help the patient age and heal at home, and the hospital actually becomes the most prohibitive cost center in that model. This was a difficult reality for many seasoned hospital executives to acknowledge. It was these mounting and increasing penalties being levied against hospitals by the Centers for Medicare & Medicaid Services CMS that eventually forced those hospitals who wanted to ignore the ACA to take action and venture into coordinated care models, joint ventures, mergers, and partnerships.

Stand-alone hospitals (not affiliated with a system) will not be a profitable business model in the future. All hospitals will need to evolve into a bigger network with a variety of services in order to survive in a value-based model, particularly stand-alone hospitals. Stand-alone hospitals must become part of an integrated delivery system and transform services to ensure that a significant portion of the systems' revenue is generated outside of the walls of the acute hospital. Hospitals that are part of a health system, ACO, BPCI, or other coordinated care initiatives that share risk and income have a significant advantage over stand-alone hospitals that have not started the transformation process.

The goal of most health systems from 2011 to 2016 was to identify new revenue streams in the post-acute and transitional care space to make up for the significant losses the organization would incur on the inpatient side as a result of reduced census and increased reimbursement audits. Remember, the ACA delivery model was designed so that organizations who successfully managed individuals' health and wellness outside of a hospital or institution would profit the most. That means that the hospital is the most prohibitive cost center in the entire business model. Will this remain true in the Trump era? That is yet to be seen but expected to be debated and picked apart for months and maybe even years after the GOP declared Obamacare dead in early 2017.

Another opportunity for health systems looking to stabilize their bottom line as a business unit of a larger organization (ACO) is to open wellness clinics or gyms targeting more mature adults. These gyms are common throughout the country and enhance and increase both physical and mental strength. A good example is the Nifty After Fifty gyms on the West Coast. Nifty After Fifty has created a rehab facility for seniors recovering from an injury that also allows the patient to continue paying privately once their insurance no longer covers the service. This allows seniors to choose a healthy lifestyle by continuing to exercise their body and mind long after recuperative therapy for the injury is complete. All else aside, this trend is one of the most glaring examples of the focus on American health care delivery shifting from a reactionary model to a model that emphasizes wellness and healthy lifestyles to reduce adverse health issues.

With all these things in mind, if the hospital is simply a cost center and the goal of the business model is to avoid the largest cost center, is there any question as to why hospitals cannot thrive as stand-alone businesses in the future? Is there any question as to why hospital operators must venture into nontraditional service lines that are self-sustaining and profitable? If a hospital census drops by 40 percent as a result of the ACA and its incentives and resources to care for patients outside of a hospital and the hospital subsequently experiences a 40 percent drop in its inpatient revenue, how does it plan to maintain the same infrastructure it once maintained in a profitable manner? Here is a simple answer: it cannot. Operating a hospital with a fee-for-service mindset in a post-ACA environment is a model that won't work. The days of the acute hospital serving as a lucrative business model are over.

Hospitals must create new revenue streams, and the business model is prioritizing outpatient and home-based services. This is exactly where the hospital must look while it still retains its power position in the continuum to create new revenue streams that can offset the forthcoming loss. It is not a model that could or might eventually evolve. The simple fact is that the legislation has already passed, and the health systems who were first to adapt have already worked through most of the growing pains. Those that did not may be looking at their final days prior to closing or being acquired. In most cases, it's inevitable.

This has been taking place for several years, and every initiative and program that was included in the ACA as well as those that were added by the CMS were designed to further promote keeping patients out of the hospital. Keeping patients well, healthy, and at home, relying on advanced technology, and a greater prioritization of living healthy is the model of the future. In this new value-based model, with so many incentives and penalties aligned against hospitals by incentivizing care outside of its setting, the days of the stand-alone hospital as a successful business model are over.

CHAPTER 7

The Unicorn Theory, ACOs, and Bundled Payment Programs

THE UNICORN THEORY

The first new program introduced by the ACA was a new alternative payment model called an accountable care organization or an ACO. As a result, the big joke in the health care profession in 2011 and 2012 went as follows:

Question: Why is an accountable care organization like a unicorn?

Answer: Because everyone knows what one looks like, but no one has ever seen one!

While I heard this stated at several health care conferences in 2011 and 2012, the reality is that in many ways, it was true. The overall census, however, is that accountable care organizations (ACOs) are just health management organizations (HMOs) by another name—a reincarnation of a managed care methodology that was very unpopular with the general public in the 1990s and 2000s. So ACOs were a reincarnation of HMOs, just with maybe a slightly different spin.

An accountable care organization is defined on the CMS (Medicare) website as follows:

> Accountable care organizations (ACOs) are groups of doctors, hospitals, and other health care providers, who come together voluntarily to give coordinated

high quality care to their Medicare patients. The goal of coordinated care is to ensure that patients, especially the chronically ill, get the right care at the right time, while avoiding unnecessary duplication of services and preventing medical errors. When an ACO succeeds both in delivering high-quality care and spending health care dollars more wisely, it will share in the savings it achieves for the Medicare program.[3]

While some would argue it is much different than an HMO of the past, if you identify the tactics for each to be successful, they are very similar.

- Deliver efficient care
- Avoid unnecessary hospitalization
- Minimize unnecessary utilization
- Communicate and coordinate between providers
- Manage high-risk patients aggressively
- Focus on keeping the patient well and healthy
- Avoid unnecessary expenditures and unnecessary procedures

While many health care executives had witnessed HMOs for many years, very few had ever seen an ACO in the flesh prior to 2012. Thus, the unicorn theory was born among the very health care leaders who were charged with the responsibility of transforming to the new model.

Fortunately, by late 2012, the unicorns flew off into the sunset as the first iteration of ACOs was launched and called Pioneer ACOs. The successes and failures of these Pioneer ACOs were shared nationally, and slowly, the industry began to learn how to effectively manage within the new regulations.

Of the thirty-two original Pioneer ACOs that existed when the program was created in 2012, by 2014, only nineteen remained as

---

[3] (https://www.cms.gov/Medicare/Medicare-Fee-for-Service-Payment/ACO/index. html?redirect=/aco; April 21, 2015)

the rest voluntarily left the program as they felt it was financially challenging.[4]

One of the main problems with ACOs when they first started was the individuals running them. Many of the original operators of ACOs were acute hospital executives who simply transferred into the ACO role. Now isn't that a backward idea? Here is a thought:

> Let's start a new business model where the entire goal is to keep patients out of the hospital and to generate savings based on finding new and efficient ways to provide quality care in the home or outside of an institutional setting. So as we start this new organization, who would be the best person to run an organization of this nature? I would argue that the last person you should look at for the job is a hospital executive or anyone who worked in a hospital environment during the fee-for-service era. However, that's exactly who was running the majority of the original ACOs. Former hospital operators who simply transferred over to the new flavor of the month business model. What a mistake that was!

Obviously, I am being facetious above, but this is an example of acute operators being the power players in the fee-for-service model and how it led to poor and defensive decisions after the passing of the ACA. Physicians were the only other group that could get a seat at the table to discuss and create new coordinated care models when the ACA was passed. Hospitals were not in the habit of engaging post-acute providers in conversation, let alone respecting their input or role as a valuable part of the care delivery team during the fee-for-service era. So naturally, many of the early ACOs were managed by either experienced acute hospital operators or physicians who were also products of the fee-for-service era and trained to gather as little information as possible on a patient and admit them to the hospital.

---

[4] (Medicare's Pioneer program down to 19 ACOs after three more exit; Evans, M.; Modern Healthcare, September 25, 2014).

Bad idea.

With that said, who would be the ideal person to manage an ACO? Would it not be someone whose background was managing costs, ensuring efficiency, and preventing unnecessary hospitalization? Perhaps a case manager or someone with a managed care background? Or maybe someone who managed a medical group during the fee-for-service era? All these roles would prepare someone to manage an ACO.

The long-standing divide between acute hospital providers, medical groups, and insurance companies led to a race among acute hospital providers to be the first to market and operate an ACO. Remember, no one knew what an ACO should look like when they were created.

Let me give you an example. I am often contacted by skilled nursing facilities who want me to help them become part of an ACO or bundle. They call and say, "Can you help us get in the hospital's ACO so we can get more of their referrals?" So in more than one instance, I actually went to the hospital to pose this question on behalf of the skilled nursing facility. The answer I was given on more than one occasion was amusing to me. I was told, "That specific skilled nursing facility is already in our ACO."

Huh? So the SNF is in the ACO, but they are not even aware, and there is no regularly scheduled care coordination meeting or phone call?

Let's just say that the first time I heard that, it gave me reason for pause. Let's go back to the basic principles of accountable care organizations for a moment. The intent is to be a coordinated care network, where providers are communicating between the different levels of care. Is that what is happening here when the convener of the ACO says, "That SNF is already contracted with our ACO," yet the SNF is not even aware they are contracted? It turns out that a lot of the ACOs just manage post-acute provider contracts in the same manner they had prior to the creation of the ACOs. Meaning, if the hospital or health system had an existing contracted rate with the skilled nursing facility in place, then the new ACO would just grandfather those contracts in for each SNF.

Does this type of approach fulfill the purpose of becoming an ACO? Absolutely not. The goal is to coordinate care one patient at a time by enhancing communication and developing a comprehensive care plan for each patient to minimize overutilization. ACOs such as the one I described above were not even including the post-acute facility in the process. Once again, it is the almighty hospital flexing that fee-for-service muscle to show "we can do whatever we want and not worry about coordinating with anyone else as we remain the 'power player.'" Time would tell that this may not exactly be the case.

Accountable care organizations were the first in a series of coordinated care initiatives all designed with the intent of encouraging providers across the continuum to communicate and innovate to improve patient care and outcomes. ACOs have come a long way in the last few years. They are certainly not the unicorns they once were. The industry now knows what a good ACO looks like as well as a poorly functioning ACO. In fact, many ACOs close up shop within a few years of opening for a multitude of reasons that led to financial failure.

It gets back to this basic principle: If health care executives were all trained as professionals during the fee-for-service era, no one would have any challenges or concerns with a value-based delivery model and patient-centered care. But since we were all trained in an era where both the provider and the physician were incentivized to institutionalize, there has been a colossal struggle to transform into a value-based model, and only in late 2015 did the industry start to see this process speed up as the federal government grew impatient with the industry's reluctance to transform.

The reality is that hospitals did not have a lot to gain from the Affordable Care Act. Whether hospitals like it or not, the fee-for-service era was a financially lucrative era for hospitals and post-acute providers. Those days are over for hospitals as the shift from volume to value is under way. It is yet to be seen how the GOP will transform the various pieces of the ACA model during the Trump era.

The Bundled Payments for Care Improvement (BPCI) program is just another attempt to get hospitals, physicians, and post-acute providers to coordinate care. BPCI programs are often referred to as "bundled payments" or "bundles." Here is the CMS (Medicare) description of the BPCI program:

On January 31, 2013, the Centers for Medicare & Medicaid Services (CMS) announced the health care organizations selected to participate in the Bundled Payments for Care Improvement initiative, an innovative new payment model. Under the Bundled Payments for Care Improvement initiative, organizations will enter into payment arrangements that include financial and performance accountability for episodes of care. These models may lead to higher quality, more coordinated care at a lower cost to Medicare.[5]

The organization selected to manage the bundle is known as the convener. These conveners are most commonly hospitals, health systems, and post-acute providers or physicians groups. The convener is the banker or insurer. Below is a more thorough explanation of a bundle awardee or convener:

> Awardees may be providers, provider networks or "conveners," defined as entities that can bring together multiple participating health care providers, such as a state hospital association or a collaborative of providers. A risk-bearing convener that also may receive payments from CMS can participate in the initiative as an awardee. A convener not able to bear risk may not receive payments from CMS but may participate in the initiative as a facilitator for participating awardee providers. Awardees will also be responsible for monitoring and reporting a variety of quality measurements to assure that appropriate levels of care are being provided. Under the initiative, an "episode" is the defined period of time during which all Medicare-covered services required to manage the

---

[5] (http://innovation.cms.gov/initiatives/bundled-payments/; April 22, 2015)

specific medical condition of a patient are grouped and paid as a unit.[6]

Although very little anecdotal data on bundles had emerged by late 2015, the CMS promoted aggressive expansion of the program. Early adopters found significant challenges in operating bundles. Specifically, bundles focus on a specific patient population that must be identified via data aggregation. Thus, almost every early adopter of bundles in 2014 struggled with early identification of the patients. In fact, many hospitals and health systems did not have the capability of aggregating this specific data even after the bundled program had begun.

Ultimately, in the bundle program, conveners must learn to ask one of the questions this book was written to promote: "How can we get this patient home with the necessary support services so they can age and heal at home?" The goal is to avoid sending patients to an SNF unless it is absolutely necessary. While originally the common perception was that these conveners would focus on shortening each patient's length of stay in an SNF, health systems quickly learned that SNF avoidance altogether was the priority if a patient was able to transfer from the hospital to be cared for at home.

Whether an ACO or a bundled payment program, the ACA introduced two new alternative payment models that reversed the trends of the fee-for-service era and mandated hospitals to employ a managed care mentality for government-paying patients. In January 2015, five years after the passing of the ACA, the CMS announced a goal of having 50 percent of Medicare patients enrolled in an alternative payment program, an ACO or a bundle, by 2018. The goal went onto say that CMS aims to have at least 90 percent of all Medicare claims tied to either quality or value by the end of 2018 as well. Unless the GOP attacks this Obama-era goal that pre-dated the Republican majority, you can expect that after 2018, the CMS will continue in the direction of requiring a higher concentration of patients being managed in an alternative payment model and

---

[6] (Staying Well within the law; Fox Rothschild Third Quarter 2011 Newsletter; Medicare Bundled Payment Initiative: Back to the Future?; March 2011).

ultimately pushing for an end to the fee-for-service era altogether. Because the underlying issue at hand in the Medicare system is the alarming rate at which funds are disappearing, a move away from this goal would be surprising even with a Republican majority as it is a major cost control preventing doctors, hospitals and other providers from providing and billing for potentially unnecessary services.

CHAPTER 8

How Do I Know if I Am in an ACO or a Bundled Payment Program?

S O NOW THAT you are an expert on alternative payment models—accountable care organizations (ACOs) and bundled payments—you are probably wondering why you have never been asked to join an ACO or a bundle. That's a good question.

You may in fact already be in an ACO. You would likely not even be aware as the means by which ACOs are formed is by enrolling physicians. If your selected primary-care physician is a member of an ACO for your insurance carrier, then you are more than likely in an ACO. How would you know? Well, I suppose you can ask. But for what reason? There is really not a significant trickle-down effect at the patient or consumer level. That is unless you have read this book or have a broad understanding of the new sophisticated alternative payment models to begin with.

If in fact you are part of an ACO, then you are less likely to fall victim to the gamesmanship and abusive practices of the fee-for-service model by a handful of physicians that placed their own financial incentives above their patients' needs and desires. If you are not already part of an ACO, if you are a Medicare recipient, it's more than likely you will be a member of an ACO by 2018.

The lingering question is this: can the Republican majority identify an alternative approach in 2017-18 to address the out-of-control spending in the delivery system by hospitals, doctors and other providers. A return to traditional fee for service with no checks and balances in-place to prevent unruly behavior by providers seems highly unlikely. There must be a system of checks and balances in place to manage the once unsustainable free-spending of Federal dollars by doctors, hospitals and other providers. These safeguards come in the form of several penalties and financial incentives for increased quality and improved communication which ultimately discourage over-utilization and prescribing of unnecessary services.

How do you know if you are in a bundled payment program? That is an even tougher question to answer. Bundled payment candidates are not "members" of a specific plan but simply Medicare participants who are assigned a specific diagnosis or procedure that has been identified by the CMS as an eligible bundled payment service. Then depending on the assigned doctor or hospital, a patient is placed into the managed bundle program for a predetermined length of time, either thirty or ninety days depending on which program you qualified for. You could be involved in a bundled payment episode and never know you were even in it!

With all this in mind, the most important factor for Americans to think about moving forward is that all payers are shifting away from fee-for-service to a managed care mentality. Managed care means limited access for patients, restrictions, required preauthorizations, and a constant messaging to live a healthy lifestyle. Thus, educating yourself on the new forms of managed care and alternative payment models is a good first step. And while it may be difficult for Medicare members to discover if they are members of an ACO or a bundled payment program at present, by the end of 2018, there will be a strong likelihood that almost all Medicare patients outside of rural areas will be assigned to an accountable care organization.

So if you are a Medicare beneficiary and want to be in the know, understand the managed care landscape and prepare for delays and required preauthorizations as the goal of the Obama Administration was to move all Medicare beneficiaries into these programs by 2020.

CHAPTER 9

Where Is All the Data?

I WALKED INTO 24 Hour Fitness a few months back for my "not so regular" weekly workout and entered my phone number on a keyboard and then scanned my fingerprint to confirm it was me. Then I walked into the gym. Wow, that was simple—modern technology. But why can't hospitals simplify in this manner?

What if each time someone walked into an emergency room anywhere in America, we had a complete medical record of that patient at our fingertips since birth? What if alongside the electronic medical record, there was a cloud-based software that also allowed input from providers, family members, and caretakers of our conversations, observations, and others pertaining to the social determinants of health care, which are often more relevant than the electronic medical record history itself?

What if it simply took a fingerprint and an identification number to access this complete personal history, or better yet, a retinal scan? Either way, it moves us closer to personalized medicine as well as instant registration and reduced wait times for patients and nonproductive time for physicians and hospitals. This is my vision for the future of health care. If 24 Hour Fitness can do it, why can't billion-dollar health care systems?

With that in mind, other questions arise. Why don't we already have more data about patients? Why don't we know more about patients when they show up in the emergency department? Why is it so difficult for health systems to get connected electronically to know more about their patients? With all the software providers and innovations available, shouldn't we be further along in terms of knowing more about an individual's health history than we do at present?

These are all valid questions. I get asked these questions a lot. The answer is simple. Hospitals have had this technology available to them for years but have chosen not to purchase it. After all, it was not conducive to their "don't ask, don't tell, just admit, then bill" approach to caring for patients in the emergency department.

In the fee-for-service era, the fact is that hospital operators did not want to know more about patients that were showing up to the emergency department. After all, if hospitals had information to prove a patient was not in fact ill or injured, then the hospital would not have been able to admit them to the inpatient floor and bill for the care delivered. Remember, heads in beds was the name of the game. Why would the hospital want to know anything more about a patient than it had to know?

Think about it this way. Hospitals have always been paid for putting heads in beds. It is a great set up for the fee-for-service era. Envision this: oftentimes, a patient shows up to the hospital, and the hospital acts like they know absolutely nothing about the patient. What a great way to justify admitting the patient so that the hospital and physician could get paid for putting a head in a bed. This scenario often happens even when the very same patient came to the hospital emergency department the day prior and had been sent home. The ineptitude of a hospital's communication on managing patients in the emergency department might be best exemplified by this hypothetical conversation:

Emergency Room Nurse A: "Hey, you do know that patient in Bed 2 was here yesterday, right?"

Emergency Room Nurse B: "Oh really, do you know who the doctor was yesterday?"

(Nurse B is assigned to the patient being discussed.)

Emergency Room Nurse A:	"Yes, it was Dr. Jones, but she is not working today."
Emergency Room Nurse B:	"Oh, well, do you know why the patient came in yesterday?"
Emergency Room Nurse A:	"No, she was not my patient. Sally was working, and she's not here today either."
Emergency Room Nurse B:	"Okay, thanks for letting me know."

That's it. That is where our desire for more knowledge ends. In the fee-for-service era, the conversation described above is about the extent that we as hospitals would go to find out as much as we could about patients who present themselves to the emergency room. This may seem laughable, but this portrays an accurate example of how our country has operated for the last thirty years.

Now let's look at the health system of the future and compare it to the conversation we described above.

Emergency Room Nurse A:	"Hey, you know that patient was here yesterday."
Emergency Room Nurse B:	"Yes, I know. When I entered her Social Security number in the computer, it popped up. There were some good notes inputted by nurse Sally yesterday. It was very helpful for me to see that the patient is complaining about the same discomfort she had yesterday, and there are no new signs or symptoms beyond what she had experienced twenty-four hours ago.

Emergency Room Nurse A:	"Interesting. She was not my patient yesterday, but today, I noticed from afar that her ankles are swollen. I'm not sure if you caught that in your assessment. You may want to check the notes to see if swollen ankles are a new development."
Emergency Room Nurse B:	"I do not recall her ankles being swollen yesterday. Let me check that out. There are some good notes in the cloud-based comments section from her daughter about adherence to our discharge directives yesterday. According to her daughter's and caretaker's input this morning, she appeared to adhere to all the directives we gave her, so we'll have to see if there's anything new."
Emergency Room Nurse A:	"Have you checked her medical record to see if she has a history of diabetes?"
Emergency Room Nurse B:	"No, I don't recall doing that, but I will do that today. Thanks for your input."

Imagine that. A world where we actually use the data that we are able to collect. Combined that with a reimbursement methodology that does not incentivize institutionalization and we may be onto something!

The hospital has always been the power player—the king of the hill. The hospital is the most influential player in the continuum and has the checkbook to make the decisions. So in a model where the hospital is paid for putting heads in beds, why would they invest in technology that could hinder their ability to admit patients? During the fee-for-service era, there was little incentive for the hospital to invest in advanced technology and electronic medical records.

The federal government put an end to that myopic mentality when they passed the ACA, including aggressive mandates for hospitals to implement electronic medical records systems. These mandates are referred to as "meaningful use" and were implemented in phases. Hospitals were penalized if they did not adhere to these deadlines. The passing of the ACA and implementation of a value-based delivery model put tremendous pressure on health systems to do the right thing by the patient in a myriad of ways.

So in short, you have these gigantic software providers and electronic medical record companies, and they send in an army of sales and tech-support people into the hospital. In most cases, they have not committed to creating a delivery model as I described above, where a lifetime of information is at the fingertips of those who need it in real time in the emergency department. Essentially, these juggernaut businesses have not accomplished even the simplest of tasks that would be in the best interest of the patient. While many health systems are getting closer to the model described above, the fact of the matter is that the technology has been there for several years, even predating the ACA in many cases. However, it simply was not the incentive of the hospitals to create that model. The January 2015 recommendation by the Department of Health and Human Services (that manages the CMS) to speed up the process of converting to coordinated care models may have been the trigger that the industry needed to start seeking a real-time alternative to secure a patient's complete medical history as well as a parallel platform for sharing information about the patient's social challenges.

The reality is, hospitals still only get paid for putting heads in beds, but all the incentives and penalties in the ACA were designed to make sure that only the right heads are put into beds. Thus, if hospitals still employ a philosophy of "find a way to justify admitting every patient we can from the emergency room," they will be penalized excessively. This is not a viable model moving forward.

CHAPTER 10

Data Blocking: The Stifling
of Innovation by Big EMR Companies

IN EARLY 2016, it appears that Andy Slavitt, the director of the
CMS at that time, had reached the same level of frustration with
the big electronic medical record (EMR) companies as the rest of the
industry. At the annual JP Morgan Healthcare Financial Summit in
San Francisco in January of 2016, Slavitt boldly proclaimed that a
change in focus for meaningful use of requirements was forthcoming
and that data blocking by EMR companies would no longer be
tolerated. He backed that up by ensuring that reduced data-blocking
and enhanced interoperability were a main focus in Washington
throughout 2016.

Data blocking? In case you are unfamiliar, as a result of the ACA's
mandates on the rapid implementation of the meaningful use of
electronic medical records, an already financially lucrative and stable
health care EMR industry became one of the strongest business
sectors in the world. The budgets for the big health system grew in
size, layers were added, and EMR became an industry within an
industry. This rapid rise to power led to a multitude of problems. The
largest of the EMR providers in the health care space grew so rapidly
that they started turning away smaller and mid-size hospitals as the
profit margin potential was not great enough.

It's pure capitalism. I lived it in the flesh when I worked within a
health system, and I have seen it time and time again and can tell you
many stories. There are two forms of data blocking that are rampant in
the health care delivery model at present. First, big EMR companies

who have long-standing, secure contracts with large health systems simply state, "Our product does not integrate with that of the doctor, post-acute facility, or other community hospital." Whether or not the big EMR company could truly integrate with these outside products is a debate in itself. It's unfathomable to me that companies this large would not have the engineers to quickly update programs to communicate and integrate.

Thus, as a result of the big EMR company's claim that its system will not integrate with the outside provider, outside providers are forced and pressured to consider shedding their existing software and buying products from the hospital's EMR company. Oftentimes, the livelihood of that physician, practice, or facility is at risk if they lose the large health system as a partner. Thus, the outside provider is forced into a corner to buy new software as a result of data blocking.

The other form of data blocking is the stifling of innovation using similar egregious business practices. In the second form of data blocking, any time a health system executive is approached by an outside vendor with an innovative solution that could benefit the hospital, improve quality, or drive cost savings, the big EMR company swoops in shortly thereafter and claims, "We offer a product that does that as well. In fact, I was advised by another hospital we service that our software probably won't integrate with that product anyway." In a sense, the new software or innovation does not even stand a chance of being adopted because as soon as they have an introductory meeting, the hospital's big EMR liaison stops by the office a few days later to brush the innovation off and say, "We can meet that need." The reality is the big EMR company rarely does follow through on the commitment to fulfill the need; their priority is more so to eliminate the threat to a portion of the hospital's IT budget that the big EMR company feels should be kept all for themselves!

I hate to be the one who breaks it to those start-up companies out there that have great concepts and innovation, but they are going to end up not winning the bid as the big EMR partner always wins. I would describe it as a tug-of-war, but it's not. It's never a tug-of-war;

it's a given. Big EMR companies will always trump the new innovator when a decision is being made by the hospital or health system.

I worked with a health system in recent years that had seven vice presidents around the table in the boardroom who reported to the CEO of the system. Who do you think was the most powerful of those vice presidents? Was it the person with the longest tenure? Was it the person who's had the most success? Was it the person responsible for quality, clinical issues, or safety? No. It was the person with the largest budget allocation. And who might that be? It is the vice president of information technology. It is capitalism. Doesn't it always work that way?

What's even more interesting, as you look around the country at the major health systems, you cannot help but notice that the health system's VP of IT is often a former employee of the EMR company that the hospital is contracted with. What a great business model for the EMR company! Some of you still might not be following me on why this is such a huge issue and why it is stifling innovation in health systems. Let me give you an example:

When a health system sets aside $4 million for its entire annual information technology budget, and they have a big EMR partner, how much of that budget do you think the big EMR partner sets its sights on for the year? Most of you probably just chuckled and said $4 million of course. I would actually beg to differ. It is more than $4 million! Let me explain.

When I worked for advertising and public relations agencies early in my career and the client set aside $4 million for advertising that year, the first thing we did was to "go back to the drawing board" and start strategizing on how we might grow that budget an additional 20 percent! Again, it's pure capitalism.

So when somebody says that the hospital sets aside $4 million for information technology this year, and the big EMR partner wants all of it, remember, this is not entirely true as they actually want all of it and more! What do you think would be the result of this? The result is that the innovative new technology available to hospitals and health systems does not stand a chance of acceptance as the health system will never invest in an outside technology as the EMR partner inevitable steps in and says, "Hey, we don't integrate with that product, but good news, we have a product that does that too!"

The reality is, even when the EMR partner has its own product that does something similar, it is usually subpar in comparison to the start-ups. This is just a means for the EMR partner to keep all the budget coming in their direction. Most of the stories I hear from health systems struggling with this issue are even worse than that. The reality is that the EMR partners often mislead their health system partners to think that they have a product which they have not actually secured yet. I have personally witnessed it on two occasions and have been advised by several others that they have had similar experiences. In my career history and in the stories I have heard, people share that their EMR partner misleads them and says that the product is in development and will be finished in the next thirty days, or they have acquired a company and are implementing. Almost every time I hear this story, six months later, the hospital partner has still been unable to meet with or speak to anyone on the other end of that product. And by that time (six months later), the team pitching the innovative solution that was originally pitched to the hospital has moved on to other potential suitors who are expressing more interest.

It is happening daily, and it is happening everywhere. It is a huge problem as it is driving the cost of health care up, yet innovation and advancement are moving at a snail's pace. The taxpayer is ultimately on the hook for this behavior by these lucrative companies. The EMR industry is thinning out as well as those powerful providers I mentioned are gaining more and more power as time goes on and their competitors fall by the wayside.

The truth is, the big EMR partners in hospitals and health systems are extremely influential, and I would argue that they are also oftentimes deceptive and sneaky. It is the almighty dollar they are chasing, and it is pure capitalism.

The acute hospital and its EMR partner are no longer the big kids on the block as they were in the fee-for-service era. But the EMR provider has found a means to stay relevant by dragging timelines out and data blocking others. For this reason, it is understandable that both are dragging their feet, but the federal government is going to see to it that these initiatives are fulfilled. It is time for health systems to start making the changes and, most importantly, do the right thing by the patient.

And finally, I have nothing against big EMR companies. The main problem I see with them is that they are trying to claim they are innovating and working with new partners all the time. The problem is, they are not listening to their hospital partners and in fact working against them in many cases. Really, can't we all just get along? We all want to make a buck, and we are all driven financially. There is, however, a mandate in this country for health systems to transform into a patient-centered, home-based delivery model. This means institutionalization of patients for health care is a last resort.

As confirmation of the narrative in this chapter, in early 2016, electronic medical record companies making up 90 percent of hospitals nationwide joined provider groups, tech giants, and health information organizations in pledging that they will not block the flow of health information between physicians and providers and agreed-upon interoperability standards. Will this commitment move the needle on the issue that has plagued health care for several years now? Many experts felt that the pledge lacked teeth and provided no consequences for those who break their promise. As a side note, both houses of Congress later passed bills punishing information blocking. Thus, accountability is coming, albeit slowly.

CHAPTER 11

Stuck on the Starting Line:
Why Can't We Just Create an Individual
Electronic Patient Record?

M Y UNDERSTANDING OF the federal government's aggressive push to implement electronic medical records in the Affordable Care Act was a desire to speed up the process of providers and physicians working together to create a personal health history or record for each individual American.

When we discussed data blocking, I shared my vision of a delivery model where all doctors and providers had access to a complete personal medical history for every patient by simply obtaining consent from the patient and entering their identification number (Social Security or another methodology). Many of the ACA-required deadlines for hospitals to implement electronic medical records referred to as "meaningful use" have already passed. With several of these meaningful use deadlines in the rearview mirror for hospitals, the assumption would be that as an industry, hospitals are a lot closer to implementing this personal health history model, would it not?

Not even close. Why, you ask? It goes back to one of the central themes of this book: It is because of capitalism, and the capitalist business owners are doing the bare minimum to meet the meaningful use requirements to avoid penalties. Few, if any of the meaningful use guidelines, have anything to do with creating a personal health history. In fact, hospitals spend almost all resources on making sure the EMR adequately addresses payment issues and the documentation required to secure reimbursement. Many call this a CYA approach—as health systems allocated all IT resources to two approaches in their efforts to avoid meaningful use penalties:

1. Implement and launch the bare minimum required to avoid penalties.
2. Focus all IT quality improvement efforts and resources on reimbursement and assuring adequate documentation is in place to secure appropriate reimbursement.

With that in mind, you can only guess as to how much progress the industry has made as a whole toward accomplishing this goal of transforming to an environment of not only creating personal health histories for individuals but also moving on to the interoperability issues of allowing a multitude of doctors and providers access to this personal history. Candidly, there has been no progress whatsoever toward this goal.

For example, you could receive care at a hospital as an inpatient for three days. A week after discharge, you could return to the emergency department of that same hospital, and more often than not, even in 2016, that hospital is not likely to have access in real time to your personal information from the stay just days prior. There is often a lag of several days. So if the same hospital is unable to access its own data for a week at a time, you can only assume how much progress has been made toward sharing such data. In most cases, unless there is a state-sponsored exchange whose sole responsibility is to drive this initiative, there has been little progress at all. Even in states with sponsored exchanges, the big health systems feel empowered to not participate or to participate on their own terms to maintain the dominant stature in the local health care delivery landscape. Like most industries, as you can see, the health care delivery system is ripe with politics at every turn.

I always wonder if anyone else sees the irony in this push for information sharing. After fifteen years of going through ridiculous measures to adhere to privacy regulations in the Health Insurance Portability and Accountability Act (HIPAA) in 1996 we have done a complete one-eighty and are now being incentivized to race toward universal electronic access to a personal patient history. Don't get me wrong, global access (with patient consent) to a universal health record (in a world free of data blocking) is absolutely the best way to ensure timely, accurate, and efficient care and achieve the triple aim of health care. With that said, the ridiculous measures that providers and physicians had to go through in order to protect patient records spiraled way out of control, and many providers used it as an excuse to not coordinate care.

Thank goodness we as a society have made the turn away from withholding pertinent information to a patient's health and are now striving to do just the opposite by creating a complete and long-term picture of the patient's health. It is not going to happen overnight, but we are starting down that road.

When President Trump appointed Dr. Tom Price to oversee the Health and Human Services role in his cabinet, the issue of interoperability and communication amongst providers in healthcare immediately reemerged as a top area of discussion. Price has been an out-spoken critic of the ACA implementation requirement deadlines for doctors and hospitals. While it is too early to know how these regulations will change, you can expect that there will be change. Let's just hope the new focus is on creating a true personal history for each patient that can be of great benefit to all providers and caretakers.

Photo Gallery

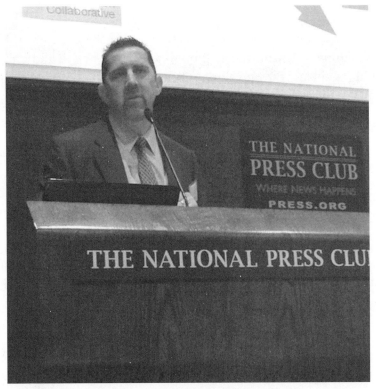

Dr. Josh Luke presents at the National Transitions of Care
Coalition annual meeting in 2015 at the National Press
Club, next to the White House in Washington DC.

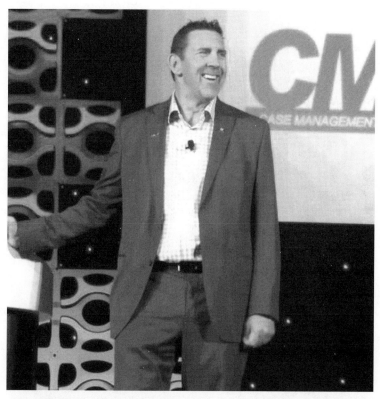

Josh Luke laughs along with the crowd as he shares a story as the keynote speaker to more than 2,500 attendees at the Long Beach California Convention Center at the annual meeting of the Case Management Society of America in 2016. Luke launched his "Discharge with Dignity" guide at the event, which is now widely accepted and used as a model in hospitals nationwide, which encourages hospitals to send patients home with support after discharge, instead of to nursing homes as has been the trend in recent years." (see guide in Chapter 25).

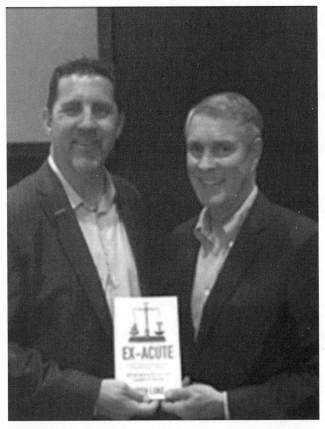

Senator William H. Frist, M.D., the Senate Majority Leader from 2002-2007, is pictured here with Josh Luke as they both were keynote presenters at an executive event in Florida in 2016.

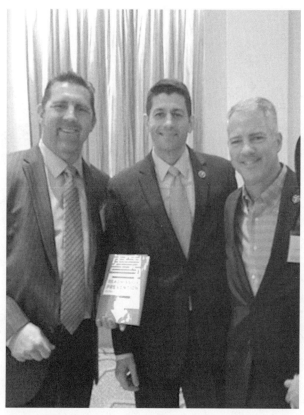

From the left: Josh Luke, House Majority Leader Congressman
Paul Ryan, and Jeff Frum from Silverado Care pose for a picture.
Luke and Ryan were both featured speakers at the Bridging
Transitions of Care event in May 2015 in Washington DC.

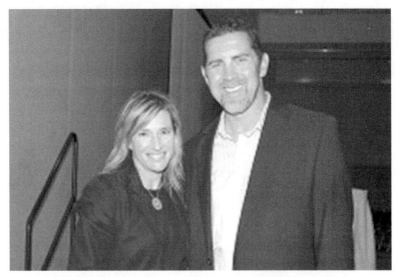

Sutter Health's Jennifer Pearce, a health literacy expert, pictured with Josh Luke after both were keynote presenters at the National Readmissions Summit in 2014.

United States Senate
WASHINGTON, D.C. 20510

November 10, 2011

Dr. Joshua Luke
Chief Executive Officer
1250 South Valley View Boulevard
Las Vegas, NV 89102-1855

Dear Dr. Luke:

Thank you for taking the time out of your busy schedule to meet with me recently.

I appreciated the opportunity to learn more about long-term acute care hospitals and your concerns about future cuts in the Select Committee process or through other legislation.

If I can be of any assistance to you in the future, please do not hesitate to contact me.

You have my best wishes.

Sincerely,

Harry Reid
United States Senator

PART 2

Lessons from the Field: Accessing Care for Your Aging Parents, Your family and Your Children

CHAPTER 12

An HMO by Another Name: Welcome to the World of Managed Care

S O WHAT NOW? First came ObamaCare, and then as soon as it started to be fully implemented Trump and the accompanying GOP majority were elected and promised to undo the ACA on day one. And while the GOP celebrated its undoing, the actual dismantling will take time. However, Accountable Care Organizations are here to stay.

If you read Part 1 of this book, then it is clear that the care we receive is the result of a screwed-up system with twisted methodologies and incentives between the patient and the provider that are not often aligned. It is becoming a managed care world, and by 2018, the jet will have firmly landed, and providers will have transition plans fully implemented to best operate a managed care business model. Managed care, in short, limits access without proper justification.

Any payer (health plan or insurance company) who reimburses physicians based on how many widgets, *errrr*, patients they see each day is seeking alternative methodologies. Almost all payers have already started this transition, and for many, it is already complete. For the federal government's Medicare program, their aggressive push will likely be in excess of 50 percent by 2018. With the exception of a few lagging and aging physicians who are set in their fee-for-service ways and have yet to retire, behaviors will change, and an entirely new mind-set for physicians and health systems will be in place by 2019. Whether or not the Obama Administration goal of having 50% of Medicare fee for service patients in an alternative payment model by 2018 lives on, the trend toward managed Medicare is likely to continue. Thus, after a year of most quality-focused hospitals and physicians managing at least half of their Medicare patients with a managed care approach in 2018, behaviors and culture will actually start to grow roots in 2019 – finally.

While Trump's GOP majority may temper the stated goal of 50% of Medicare being managed by 2018, it is the inevitable result of transformation necessary to manage remaining Medicare funds efficiently. All politics aside, the Federal Government will finally have some spending controls in place to limit the laissez-faire approach providers adopted in the 1980's and 1990's, and continued after the millennium. Frankly, it should never have taken this long. The GOP majority will lead to an aggressive expansion of Medicare Advantage programs in coming years as well.

To best clarify the above statements, it is important for the reader to understand two key principles about care delivery in the emergency room:

1) Prior to examining a patient and providing care, hospitals and doctors are not permitted legally to ask if the patient has insurance or who their insurance provider is.
2) Thus, hospitals and doctors must approach all patients in the emergency room in the same manner as they are unaware if the patient is managed care or not.

As a result of these regulations, overutilization (ordering several often-unnecessary labs or tests) of patients became the norm during the fee-for-service era. This was a result of several factors:

1) Liability. Doctors would rather be safe than sorry. And hey, why not, we all get paid more if we order more tests!
2) Relationships, nepotism, or quid pro quo. Call it what you want, but doctors adhere to the "you scratch my back (financially), and I will scratch yours in return." The more tests that were ordered, the more doctors got involved and billed.
3) Justification. Let us not forget the almighty quest for justification, in any way shape or form, to admit an emergency department

patient to the hospital. We must go fishing for at least some medical reason to back it up! Heads in beds, whatever it takes.

Fast forward to forty years of creating and implementing these habits, and in 2018, the payer world is turned upside down. No more widgets to bill for, no more heads in beds reimbursement, no more reward for volume- and quota-based physicians. It's a managed care world now. And all patients, seniors in particular, in 2018 and beyond must be treated as managed care, whether they are or not.

The truth about 2018 is that it will effectively mark the end of the fee-for-service era as we know it, regardless of if the name sticks. The reality is even in what we refer to as traditional Medicare fee for service, there are so many new penalty and incentive programs for doctors, hospitals and other providers, that even the traditional fee for service product is significantly value based. These penalties focus on quality factors, criteria based decision making, infection rates, avoidable readmission rates and referral patterns for post acute care among other topics.

In fact, Trump's appointee to oversee the Center for Medicare and Medicaid Services, Seema Verma, has traditionally supported patient penalties if they are using the emergency department and other resources unnecessarily. So these financial penalties and accountability measures are not just targeting doctors and providers, but patients as well – touche'! Accountability for all!

Many providers and physicians are still struggling to see how they will fit in, which is completely understandable. This transition is done in the name of more effective, patient-centered care. The federal government loosely translates patient-centered care as an approach that focuses more on the patient and less on how physicians and providers are reimbursed. Another common cliché is "from volume to value." That simply means we are making a shift from a widget-based (volume) reimbursement methodology to a value-based methodology that rewards physicians and providers for reducing utilization (testing, appointments, etc.).

Whether you are a hospital operator, a home health agency or SNF owner, or a doctor, I have one last word for those fee-for-service holdouts as we approach 2018, and readers can feel free to join in with me in saying it out loud if it has not been made clear yet: "Fee-for-service as we knew it (in the good old days for doctors and hospitals) is dead!" The Federal Medicare fund is soon to be empty. Are you prepared?

America is rapidly becoming a completely managed care environment for health care. It's a managed care world, and we're just living in it!

CHAPTER 13

A Mother's Guide to Accessing Quality Care for Her Family in a Managed Care World

REMEMBER, THE *"BETTER. SMARTER. Healthier."* goal established by the federal government in January 2015 aimed to have more than 50 percent of the Medicare hospital claims (invoices) within an alternative payment model (ACO or bundle) by 2018. Unless the Trump Administration reverses this goal, which seems likely at some level, this means that operationally hospitals will strategically attempt to ensure more than 70 percent of their key physicians are enrolled in an ACO.

By announcing this goal, this served as a forceful push and a shot-across-the-bow to providers if you will, to expect additional penalty programs from the CMS in the near future, especially if the CMS perceives that the transition to alternative payment models is not being done proactively by providers. This goal by the CMS is one that has been applauded by yours truly to prompt more timely responses from hospitals and other providers in converting to alternative payment models (or managed care).

Due to changes in care delivery behavior as a result of these care coordination mandates, by 2018, it is likely that hospitals will be treating all patients like managed care patients, which translates to more efficient and timely care. Something seems to be working! However, Tom Price, Trump's appointee to lead Health and Human Services was an outspoken critic of mandated alternative payment models (like ACO's and bundles) during the Obama Administration. Thus, it is likely that this goal will be extended or adjusted in 2017-18.

So for those of you more comfortable with numbers than words, let's convert this formula into a math equation:

Alternative Payment Models (APM) = Accountable Care Organization (ACO) or Bundled Payment

ACO or Bundle = Managed Care

Managed Care = HMO (Health Maintenance Organization)

Thus, APMs = HMOs

So how do you approach a managed care world? Managed care limits access unless accompanied by justification and appropriate documentation. Thus, here are a few key tactics to approaching managed care that all mothers seeking to access quality care for their families should understand:

- Educate yourself and understand the system
- Prepare for delays
- Expect required preauthorizations
- Do not expect to be hospitalized when you visit the emergency department, unless your situation is clearly emergent
- Ask lots of question
- Be empowered to question every care decision, if for clarity if nothing else
- Understand home-based technology
- Be prepared for increased self-management of conditions and accountability
- Be persistent

So let's talk about that last bullet point. Guess what? The squeaky wheel wins even in health care. What do I mean by that? Humans are well, human. When the phone of the scheduler of the doctor's office rings every morning at 9:01 a.m. with the same request from the same individual, for an approval of an appointment, the scheduler is likely to approach the decision maker and advocate for an approval. If only life were that easy! Well, in some cases, actually in many cases in health care, it can be that simple if you are willing to be persistent.

Be prepared to learn about operating home-based technology as well. Self-management will be a new theme that emerges. Imagine that? Americans actually taking some responsibility for their own health! Home-based technology is rapidly being proven to be a cost-efficient means to save health care dollars and improve health, but it often requires the patient being educated on how to self-administer the technology.

I am a Gen-Xer, and I loved the eighties. Thus, I just cannot end this chapter any other way but to pay tribute to Madonna by creating a theme song for moms looking to best access health care for their families in a post-ACA environment: "We are living in a managed care world, and I must be a managed care girl . . ."

Read on.

CHAPTER 14

A Lesson in Capitalism: Why Your Family's Health Care Costs Will Continue to Increase

THE COST OF accessing health care in America will continue to rise. It's a certainty.

Regardless of who won the Presidential election in 2016, one fact is assumed: health care delivery costs will continue to increase. Thus, the cost of insuring your family and maintaining your family's health will continue to increase as well. There is a short answer as to why, as well as a more detailed explanation. I will provide you both in this chapter. First, let's discuss the short answer as to why health care costs in America will continue to rise for the foreseeable future.

Its capitalism, deal with it.

Well, you are probably entitled to a longer answer than that, but it's a capitalistic society we live in, and with change comes opportunity. Everyone is trying to make a buck. Don't blame the messenger, whether Republican or Democrat, whether proponent or opponent of the Affordable Care Act.

Remember that the ACA had a triple aim: improved care, better health, and less cost (efficiency). Thus, President Obama's goal with Obamacare to reduce costs may have ultimately come to fruition had ObamaCare survived. But not in this decade. There are too many iterations, innovations, transitions, transformations, implementations, technological mandates and leadership changes to get it all right so quickly.

This is especially true with a GOP majority behind President Trump, as the entire delivery system will be scrutinized and tweaked piece by piece. Remember, getting the ACA passed was said to be President Obama's top goal when he was elected. He sought out to make healthcare reform his primary legacy. Looking back, in a twisted way, healthcare reform and its undoing after he left office may ultimately be his lasting legacy.

The most significant political mistake made by President Obama in his rush to get the ACA passed was that he created much of it through executive orders that required only his signature, and not a vote of Congress. While this may have seemed logical at the time as Democrats were largely in support of the legislation, anything created with just the signature of an executive order can be undone just as easily with the signature of a new President. In comes Trump, whose campaign promise was to undo ObamaCare on Day one in the White House. And all it could have taken was the stroke of an ink pen, but Congress passed the repeal in both houses even prior to inauguration day.

So let's take a closer look at some of these technologies and innovations and why it's taking so long for them to have the desired effect on healthcare delivery. Look no further than electronic medical records. When the ACA was passed, it passed a series of requirements for hospitals and physicians to implement software and electronic medical records on a short timeline. Do you think that led to lower prices and increased competition? Of course not! It led to price gouging, monopolistic tactics, excessive data blocking, and arrogant, deceptive, and misleading business practices from the leading EMR companies. Why? Because they could!

Within a few short months, several big EMR companies were turning away small and medium-size hospitals as the "account was not big enough to bother with unless you are part of a larger health system." While change may bring opportunity, it did not guarantee innovation or progress in a timely manner when it came to technology. And costs shot through the roof as a result. Again, these costs are passed on by hospitals and doctors to payers and families. All in the name of capitalism!

Additionally, a number of the new penalty and incentive programs not only cater to third-party assisting doctors, hospitals, and payers but also require third parties to administer the programs. Bundled payments are a great example. These large "convening" consulting firms became very powerful in a short amount of time. One, naviHealth became so powerful in such a short amount of time by servicing bundled payment programs for large organizations like Dignity Health and others that it was bought out in August 2015 by Cardinal Health, one of the largest medical suppliers in the country. It acquired 71 percent of naviHealth for approximately $290 million.

$290 million for a third-party consulting firm? Wow. That's capitalism at its finest. What if the feds come back and discourage the use of third parties by incentivizing health systems and providers to do this on their own? Well, that's a realistic option as the Medicare Payment Advisory Commission members at their December 2015 meeting were almost unanimous in striking down a new post-acute reform measure that required a third party. The overwhelming message from the commissioners, who make recommendations to the federal government on changes to the Medicare system, was that all the dollars being allocated to health systems and hospitals for effectively coordinating care seem to be getting passed directly to third parties.

Thus, there really is no financial incentive in many ways for health systems and hospitals to improve coordinated care efforts. Beware of the third-party provider, the tide may be turning. However, I am confident that naviHealth and Cardinal have done an admirable job diversifying to make their services needed, as they were likely the first to see this potential shift away from simple conveners coming!

There are so many middlemen in health care that it is difficult to keep up. Look at supplies for example. In order to adequately care for a patient, the supply process may go like this:

Raw materials acquired by manufacturer	→	Hard cost
Manufacturer creates product/device	→	Hard cost
Manufacturer sells wholesale to medical supplier/distributor	→	Hard cost
Distributor secures delivery from trucking company	→	Hard cost
Hospital pays materials management staff to inventory	→	Salary
Central supply stocks hospital/operating room shelf	→	Salary
Nurse/physician administer product	→	Salary
*Many devices require a manufacturer's trained rep in the room	→	Hard cost
Physician bills for application	→	Insurer billed
Hospital bills insurer for product and application of product	→	Insurer billed to cover all

Those are the ten steps to get a device to a patient. Each comes with a cost. That cost is ultimately passed on to you.

One of the inherent issues with personal health care costs is that the health insurance industry is one of the few industries in the country that has a third party negotiating an individual's costs. Think about it, you don't have a third party with you at the car dealership when negotiating a car price. You negotiate directly. Negotiation is not just an art that requires intelligence. It is a very emotional process as well. When you go to Walmart or Target, do you bring a third party with you to negotiate prices? No. But when necessary, you exercise the ultimate negotiating tactic and walk away when a store increases its prices to a level you are not comfortable with.

Why the middleman in health care? Is an insurance company even necessary?

Have you seen the annual compensation packages of managed care executives and health system executives? They are not poor. One insurance CEO took home more than $17 million in 2013. Can I just ask a common sense question? Is that really necessary? $17 million a year? I bet that's not the insurer's first message point on the agenda at the annual member town hall meeting! It might be the member's first agenda item though! $17 million? That's like winning the lottery to most. Imagine if that $17 million were split up among its global members in the form of a rebate check? Wow, that could be a few bucks per member at a minimum!

While I am all for capitalism and the free market, at some point, some of these few very fortunate executives need to get a little closer to reality and understand how that message feels to a member who is struggling. And this goes for health system executives as well. Everyone is entitled to make a living, and yes, there is great responsibility in these roles, but there are other ways to protect an individual from liability and these responsibilities than simply compensation. The federal government should be applauded for attempting to include safeguards in the ACA to limit the spending and compensation of insurers, but it's a task that's much easier said than done.

Any way you look at it, some of the executive compensation packages in health care do not feel good to the struggling single mom or middle-class family just trying to raise a healthy family.

CHAPTER 15

Should I Check Out a High-Deductible Insurance Plan?

T HE PASSING OF the Affordable Care Act brought the return and rapid emergence of high-deductible insurance plans for many families. Some families had no choice. If they wanted health insurance, then the high-deductible plan is the only one with monthly costs that fit into the budget. Even with Trump in the White House, high deductible plans are likely to stay, and may even grow in popularity as he is a proponent of the free market and consumers right to choose.

A high-deductible plan works like this. Your monthly costs for insurance are lower, but if a family member is hospitalized or needs care (often referred to as an "episode" of care), the bulk of the initial costs will be your responsibility. Thus, your insurance does not actually start paying for any of the costs of the episode of care until you have contributed to the deductible amount, oftentimes $2,500 or $5,000. For example, in addition to your monthly payment, the first $5,000 spent on care that calendar year is the responsibility of the individual. In this scenario, if the monthly premium was $400 ($4,800 annually) and the deductible was $5,000 annually, then the first $9,800 of care that year would be the individual's responsibility and not paid for by the insurer. In return, the insurer has contracted for "preferred rates" with providers for you to pay less.

However, you would still get access to those preferred rates in a more traditional plan, which may be structured more like this: Your monthly premium is $600 ($7,200 annually), but your annual deductible is only $1,000. In this scenario, your annual costs would be less, totaling

$8,200 for the year. However, if you are an individual who rarely needs care, then the high-deductible plan could cost you significantly less than $9,800 annually as you are only required to spend the monthly premium of $400, and in a healthy year, your costs may not exceed $4,800 if you access no services.

High-deductible plans are becoming a target of more and more scrutiny because they are often purchased by families and individuals who do not likely have the means to cover the deductible if in fact the member became ill or injured. Oftentimes, high-deductible plans may be episode based as opposed to a minimum spending threshold for the year. If you are hospitalized, then you are responsible for the first $2,000, and the insurer may pay the balance or a portion thereof.

There are several new alternatives to high-deductible policies. When shopping for insurance for yourself or your family, you should research your options thoroughly. In addition to high-deductible policies, the ACA brought drastic change to who qualifies for federal assistance and what requirements an employer has in providing insurance benefits.

This will be ever-changing but one thing that is certain is that access to care was the cornerstone of the ACA. As a result, access will continue to be under the microscope during the Trump Administration. The end result is likely to be a level of access to care to the middle class that is significantly broader than in the pre-ACA era when Obama took office. How that looks remains to be seen, but increased access (over the pre-ACA options) even after the ACA repeal is likely.

Among the emerging trends are co-op insurance plans. Many compare them to credit unions as they evolved out of existing groups or organizations that realized by co-opting funds, they could create large enough pool to cover everyone's health costs. This is only true if everyone acts responsibly of course. One of the most successful co-ops nationwide is Medi-Share, found online at *www.MyChristianCare.org*.

My brother approached me a few years ago, as after the passing of the ACA, his small-business PPO (preferred provider organization) insurance plan notified him that his costs were increasing by more than 200 percent as a result of the mandated changes in the ACA. I told him I had dealt with co-ops in my days as a hospital CEO but always treated them just like insurance companies. Since then, my brother joined the co-op, lowered his costs in comparison to his pre-ACA premiums, and thought it was wonderful.

Most importantly, do your research when shopping for a policy for yourself and your family. With all these in mind, let's think back to the prior chapter on capitalism and in the next chapter discuss some tactics to help those of you who are in a high-deductible plan or even just those who want some insights on how to reduce your health care costs. Hint: remember the mention of the squeaky wheel and being persistent.

CHAPTER 16

How to Save a Few Bucks When You Access Care: Getting Discounts from Doctors and Hospitals

W HEN YOU GET a hospital bill in the mail, or a physician bill for that matter, does it often look like it was written in another language? Or better yet, does it look more like a math problem on a high school Algebra test? Someone ought to write a book called "Paying Medical Bills for Dummies," and I will put a down payment on the first copy right now. Heck, I was a hospital CEO for almost ten years and have no idea how to translate a hospital bill when it comes in the mail!

Have any of you ever paid a medical bill only to find out later that you paid too soon, as the insurer had not yet paid? I have. If you are struggling financially, have lost a job or need a longer period of time to pay medical bills, following are some tips that may help. Keep in mind, health insurance is one of the only industry's in a capitalistic society like the United States where a third party is empowered to negotiate pricing on an individual's behalf. Empower yourself to negotiate these bills and occasionally the hospital or doctor may agree as in many cases it is mutually beneficial.

Guide to Saving Health Care Dollars and Paying Hospital Bills

1. Negotiate in advance with the provider (doctor or hospital) when possible. Co-pays, deductibles, procedure costs, all of

the above! Its money, and it's yours . . . until you give it to them, then it's gone.

    a.   This is especially true for elective procedures

        i.   Non-emergent surgeries, procedures, or tests
        ii.   Cosmetic surgeries
        iii.   Orthodontics
        iv.   Dental procedures

2. When a bill arrives in the mail from a hospital, physician, or dentist, either call them or hold the bill for one month before paying to confirm insurance has paid and any applicable preferred provider discounts have been applied. Keep it to compare against the next month's copy. Hospitals and doctors generate invoices monthly, so save them to compare. You are sure to learn a lot!

3. Reference against your explanation of benefits (EOB) from your insurance company and personal health portal (when available; more on this in the Technology chapter) to confirm appointment dates and procedures.

4. After one month has gone by and after comparing all documents, call the provider to confirm the amount on the most recent invoice is accurate as it often takes one to two bill cycles for insurance payments to post and discounts to be applied to the bill. If you pay before this takes place, you may in fact be overpaying your responsible portion.

5. Confirm with the provider if insurance has in fact paid or not. If not, are they expecting insurance to pay, and has there been any communication to confirm?

6. When the amount is reasonable, pay the bill over the phone using your debit or credit card and appropriately allocate it for your tax records.

Bonus! Empower yourself to request a discount from the provider for any amount over $200, especially if the amount is over $1,000!

So let's talk about this bonus bit of information. It's an inherent trait in a capitalistic society, and few individuals choose to exercise it in health care. For doctor bills that are in excess of a few hundred dollars, I suggest appealing to the personal side of the billing person on the other end of the phone. Call them and let them know.

Believe it or not, getting hospitals to offer significant discounts is easier than in the doctor's office, as the doctor's office has a much thinner margin and less cash flow. Just have your credit card ready to go while you are on the call! The hospital and its staff understand that a single payment of $200 is difficult for an individual on any monthly budget to afford, and they also understand that the alternative is that you may not pay at all. The fact that you called them to discuss it is satisfying to them, as a large part of their jobs as collectors is to simply get people on the phone to discuss the outstanding debt.

I will let you in on a little secret. Your outstanding 90-day bill is so irrelevant to the hospital in the bigger picture. Hospitals sell their receivables to third parties (there is the third party again), who pays ten cents on the dollar to the hospital for outstanding deliverables. That third party gets to keep everything they collect. And you bet the third party employs the tactics of a collection agency!

With this in mind, that they are selling your bill after 180 days unpaid, at ten cents on the dollar to Guido, someone's Italian cousin who employs stronger telephonic collection tactics than a hospital prefers to, it makes a lot more sense as to why a hospital will waive up to 50 percent of a bill when you have a credit card in hand. It is not a perfect art, but it is worth a shot. After all, it is your money. The worst thing that could happen when you request a discount is the provider simply saying no. And then your right back where you started and there is nothing lost in the process. Remember, sometimes the provider or doctor may be cash poor when you ask and actually prefer giving you a discount to get money in the door, as an alternative to you making monthly payments.

Since this is the chapter where I usually aggravate physicians altogether and they either put the book down for good and don't finish reading it, or go online to write a scathing review (hey, scathing reviews sell books!), let me share a few facts with you that provide justification for the need for a chapter on attempting to get discounts from hospitals:

- Ultimately, the hospital and physician are under no obligation whatsoever to offer you any discount.
- 2016 represented the first year that an individual American's health care costs eclipsed $10,000 annually. For a family of five, $50,000 eclipses the national average household income altogether.
- Remember, health insurance is one of the only examples in a capitalistic society like the United States where a third party is empowered to negotiate pricing on an individuals behalf.
- In July 2016, Congress passed strict debt collection rule changes that drastically changed how hospitals and other businesses can pursue health care debt from consumers.

One last editorial note on this topic. I recently called a local doctor to see if he could fit my wife in for an appointment that same afternoon. The receptionists at his office answered the phone and her response to my question was not "yes or no," but "do you have an HMO or a PPO?" Just to be clear that I heard her correctly, I asked the same question again. "I was calling to see if the doctor would be able to see my wife this afternoon?" She replied with the same answer the second time I asked. This financial approach is a two way street as you can see from her response.

But remember, we are all human and have the right to appeal to their human side. But be nice when you call, not rude or snippy! You are making an emotional appeal, human to human so put yourself in their shoes and consider how you would best be approached.

That high-deductible plan may not be sounding so bad anymore, heh?

CHAPTER 17

How Can My Family Utilize Technology to Increase Access to Quality Health Care?

TECHNOLOGY. IT'S EVERYWHERE we look in health care. But where do we start?

First, technology will play a key role in everyone's personal health moving forward as self-management will become a central focal point for insurers, whereas traditionally, insurers relied on patients to manage their own medication. Beyond medication, management patients were advised to go visit a doctor or clinic.

Advancements in technology have changed this. Patients are able to read and apply tests in the home that previously required a trained nurse or doctor. And guess what? Oftentimes, the patient does not even need to report the outcome of a daily test as the outcome is wirelessly transmitted to the insurer's database and care manager. If the result shows to be high risk or an outlier of sorts, an alarm message notifies the insurer, and the care manager initiates contact with the patient or physician to best meet that need.

For example, many insurance companies now provide scales to seniors. Seniors can now weigh themselves on their own in their home instead of daily visits to a doctor or clinic when recovering. The scale uses wireless technology to update the database and alert the caretaker of the result. If their daily weight gain exceeds normal limits, an alarm is triggered, and the caretaker contacts the patient to discuss the situation.

In fact, self-management has become so prevalent in recent years that there are many humorous stories about how difficult it can be to actually get an accurate weight reading from a patient self-administering. One insurer relayed to me that the patient's weight was down twelve pounds one day from the day prior. When the care manager initiated contact, the patient revealed that she was leaning on the table during the weigh-in as she did not want to fall over as she was watching *Oprah*. Another patient reported that her weight had increased eighteen pounds in one day. The truth turned out to be that she guessed at her weight (which in this case was prewireless technology) and advised the caretaker later that she guessed as there was no one there to help her, and she could not read the scale as she did not have her glasses on. Who said there is no humor in health care!

More commonly, we are seeing bracelets. Fitbit is one example that can give an individual a fairly accurate reading of their activity for the day as well as their heart rate. This personalized technology continues to evolve rapidly to help individuals better understand how to improve their own health and to alert when warning signs are setting in.

Likewise, there are diet applications that can assist an individual in understanding what they are eating, including calories, carbohydrates, fat and sodium. With all the diet fads that come and go each year, these apps and software provide individuals the opportunity to track their intake of each of these key indicators or weight gain, loss, or overall health. The days of focusing just on calorie intake or carbohydrate intake are going away as most of these applications like "Lose It" illustrate each on the same screen and alert you when one category is excessive.

A few additional new trends are the connectivity capabilities of physicians, hospitals, care takers, patients and family members. The ACA brought the mandating of personal patient portals. Many individuals already have a personal health website that tracks appointments, bills, referrals, and test results and is usually connected to resources to educate and improve self-management. Active use of a personal patient portal can be extremely beneficial. With the easy accessibility of mobile phones and applications, millennials and future generations will likely adapt quickly to using a personal health portal and will likely become a mainstream societal practice within a few short years.

While hospitals communicated via technology with encrypted text messaging through an organization called Tiger Text in the 2000s, since then, organizations like MediGram and others have developed secure messaging platforms that allow other individuals to opt in to the dialogue pertaining to an individual's care. I call this a "cloud-based parallel" or "personal health vine" to the electronic medical record that allows personal input from caretakers and family members. A patient can consent to allow anyone access to his or her "vine," and it simply is a chat room in which a physician posts instructions, caretakers can respond or ask questions, family members can chime in, pharmacists can provide instructions, and the patient himself can engage as well.

Remember the conversation earlier about the emergency department of the future? A world in which you show up to the hospital and the emergency department doctor has access not only to your complete medical history but also to your private health vine (more formally referred to as your cloud-based health care data). Oftentimes, it is input from a family member or caretaker that proves to be much more valuable to an emergency department physician than anything a personal medical history can illustrate.

To provide an example, let's hypothetically discuss Jim, a middle-aged patient who lives at home with his spouse, Emily. Jim sits on the couch all day and watches television as he quit working because of a leg injury the prior year. He has not been able to find work since he has recovered from this injury. In recent weeks, Jim reports to Emily that he has extreme back pain every afternoon between 2:00 p.m. and 3:00 p.m. Jim is not a great communicator, verbal or electronically, so Emily enters the time and severity as well as the location of the pain every day into Jim's personal health vine.

After a week of this pain, they decide to go visit Jim's doctor, who is unable to identify a serious problem other than soreness because of lack of exercise, being overweight, and lack of physical activity. The next week, Emily travels out of town on a three-day business trip and hires a caretaker to watch Jim for four hours a day in their home. Jim complains to the caretaker of back pain between 2:00 p.m. and 3:00 p.m. on the first day and again on the second day. On the second day, the caretaker wants to play it safe, so she takes Jim to the hospital. Once at the hospital, the emergency room doctor reviews any medical history that the hospital has on Jim in the electronic medical record, sees no history of back pain, and runs a number of tests. The hospital does not have access to the doctor's notes from the prior week's office visit as the big EMR company that works with the hospital did not feel it was enough of a priority to connect the doctor (there was not enough profit in it for them). Neither Jim nor the caretaker informs the doctor that the pain has been building over a few weeks, and neither advises the emergency doctor of the personal health vine.

After Jim and the caretaker have spent six hours in the emergency department, Emily returns home and finds that Jim and the caretaker are at the hospital waiting for test results. Emily shows up at the hospital, worried, only to find the reason for the trip was the same back pain as days prior. The doctor then returns with nothing to report and encounters Emily who reports the prior week's doctor visit and the vine that shows the back pain has been constant for several weeks, and two Advil usually solves the problem. "I wish I would have known. I would not have run all those expensive tests," the doctor says in reply. Emily proceeds to advise him that all that information had been recorded in Jim's personal health vine that was accessible via his mobile phone or any local computer. The doctor answers, "Jim never mentioned that he had a personal health vine, and had I seen that information, I would have sent him home with two Motrin five hours ago!"

So there is an example of how the cloud-based conversation parallel or personal health vine can prove to be much more valuable than an electronic health record that is not so much about your health and history but more so focused on documentation to justify payment by the insurer.

How does an individual access this personal health vine? The easiest way is to create a group message in your mobile phone. However, the smarter, more secure, and HIPPA-compliant method is to wait until your insurer offers you the product they offer for this purpose.

Technology is available to improve your health and your access to health. Thus, if you have a great desire to utilize technology for this purpose, do a little research and there is likely a solution of some sort out there for you and your family.

CHAPTER 18

Millennial Culture: Wellness
and Healthy Lifestyles

REMEMBER JUST A few years ago when the word "wellness" came with connotations of Eastern medicine and a physician office lobby with calming water fountains, harmonious instrumentals, and an aroma filling the air reminiscent of a fully bloomed flower garden? Not anymore. Wellness and healthy lifestyles are one of the most common traits of our youngest generations.

While GenXers like myself brought a pattern of unhealthy issues such as poor dietary choices and a lack of activity that led to problems associated with obesity, as millennials become the target of Madison Avenue, technology that enables healthy decisions in real time is available, affordable, and accessible to everyone. As a result, it has become much easier to make healthy decisions. Thus, dietary habits are improving, and fitness is becoming more of a priority.

As a result of health care reform, this trend will only be even more so true. The ACA actually had a number of initiatives that provide financial incentives for health care providers and employers whose workforce made healthier decisions. As a result, improved health led to better care at a lower cost. Sound familiar? It should, as you recall those are the three pillars of the triple aim of health care reform.

So wellness is no longer simply a luxury for the wealthy; it is synonymous with living a healthier lifestyle. Many employers have invested in workplace fitness and health incentive programs and reward employees for making wise decisions that lead to better health. These programs offer rewards, similar to credit card points or frequent flier miles, for making healthy decisions such as quitting smoking, increasing exercise or steps daily, reducing body fat ratio, and eating healthier foods. It's important to note that these programs don't necessarily just reward that fitness fanatic that sits in the office next to you at work and carries her own water bottle with her each day (often with some odd-colored concoction that we are told is some type of unique formula that burns body fat mysteriously!). These programs reward everyone equally, and it is often the individual with the worst habits who shows improvement and can benefit the most in the long run—both in life and in rewards points!

Similar to employers emphasizing health and wellness, some universities are taking the same approach. In the fall of 2015, Oral Roberts University (ORU) in Tulsa, Oklahoma, began requiring all incoming freshmen to wear Fitbits. Although ORU has required students to track fitness for several years, 2015 marked the first year that students at the institution fulfilled ORU's required commitment to "mind, body, and spirit" by tracking bodily activity electronically.[7] Each student's heart rate and number of steps walked are electronically reported to an instructor, and the results account for approximately 20 percent of the student's physical fitness grade. What a great example of how technology is opening doors for millennials that no other generation has had the luxury of benefitting from in their teen and college years.

Another example of this transition to healthy lifestyles is the gyms that are popping up nationwide, catering to the middle-aged and the baby boomer generation. These gyms are often outpatient rehabilitation facilities that also serve as long-term workout facilities for aging adults. Although the insurer often pays for the first few weeks of recovery and rehab in these facilities, the gyms were created so that individuals can pay privately to continue coming even when they are back to full health (a twenty-four-hour fitness for seniors). One example of this is in Southern California. Dr. Sheldon Zinberg, founder of Caremore,

---

[7] Modern Healthcare, January 2015 page 36. "Fitness trackers aren't elective at Oral Roberts University."

created the concept of Nifty-After-Fifty, a gym designed specifically for seniors. The concept has been so successful that other medical groups and insurers have joined together to invest in these facilities that double as both outpatient medical rehab facilities and fitness gyms for those who are fully recovered.

These gyms don't just have equipment for physician health but also have computers that test and stimulate mental and cognitive growth. Many of these facilities also have dietitians, occupational therapists, nurses, physical therapists, and other skilled health care workers on-site for a few hours every week to provide access and support to members.

It's a genius idea when you think about it. The medical insurer, who is financially responsible for your health, is creating an environment that you pay for privately and separately to improve your health. It becomes a desired social routine for many as well as an integral part of their lifestyle. It's a senior center for active seniors—just don't tell the individuals working out there that they are seniors!

On that note, one thing you will learn working in health care is that no one thinks they are old or sick. If you have not yet learned that from your grandfather or grandmother, you learn it quickly when you work in the senior health care space. No one thinks they are old. It is human nature. Do you know how many years my grandmother could be heard saying, "I am the youngest person living in this retirement community. The rest of them are old"? She said that right up until her death in her mid-eighties (Bless her heart!). But let's do the math here. It's a senior community that required all residents be sixty or older. And she lived there for twenty years! So while it may have been true that she was one of the younger folks when she moved in, it turns out I was the typical gullible grandchild who twenty years later was still believing her when she would take me to the shuffle board park and tell me she was the youngest resident in the park! Looking back, fat chance of that being true in her eighties!

Let me give you a similar example of that mind-set in health care. I worked at several multilevel senior communities through the years.

On these campuses, there are typically independent living apartments, assisted living apartments, a memory care unit and a skilled nursing facility (often called the health center), as well as a physician's office and a rehab area. The residents convene in the dining room three times a day, in the activities room and garden in-between, and take periodic trips on the shuttle to the store, mall, casino, and ball game or on outings. However, when a patient falls ill or gets injured and is taken to the hospital, and then the doctor advises them they need additional care in a nursing home before they return to their independent or assisted living apartment, the residents all refuse and insist on staying in the hospital until they can be discharged straight home.

Why? Well, it is likely just plain human nature. But the residents will tell you that the health center (nursing home) on campus is "where the old folks who are sick stay." Others will suggest "that is where the older residents go to die." So it's a perception that is common among the generation.

All this considered, it is likely that insurers will start providing additional financial incentives to patients who live healthier lifestyles. While the current trend is to reward with incentives such as gift cards and electronics in these workplace fitness programs, it is likely that regulations will begin allowing insurers more liberty in returning cash discounts to patients who commit to healthy lifestyles and consent to electronic monitoring to prove it. Sound familiar? It's the same approach that auto insurers have been taking to discount auto rates for years. The health care insurers are slower to market as health care is one of the most highly regulated industries in the world, and health care finance is no exception to those stringent regulations.

Qualcomm and UnitedHealth announced a program in early 2016 called United Healthcare Motion that gives enrollees in United insurance plans wearable devices that have the ability to track how many steps they take each day. Employees who use the devices can earn up to $1,460 per year in savings, which will be placed in a health savings account. The transformation to healthier lifestyles supported by corporations (who are paying high premiums for health insurance) has begun!

CHAPTER 19

Millennials: Don't Look Now but They Are Running Your Hospital

S O WITHOUT SOUNDING like a research geek, let me share some common traits of the millennial generation in the health care space based on my experiences and education. We know that millennials are tech savvy and therefore can multitask. Being tech savvy has also programmed their generation to value instant gratification and connectivity. But in their careers more specifically, millennials seek transparency and advancement.

Well, they might just get their wish.

While I was fortunate to become a hospital CEO at age thirty-two, I was one of the few GenXers who was able to reach the head role within a hospital. While the number 2 and 3 positions within many organizations were often GenXers themselves, there was very little turnover and succession planning in the hospital sector in the 1990s and 2000s, the heyday of the fee-for-service era—a time when hospitals were generating huge profit margins nationwide. If you are a CEO, why retire? Hospital executives were pulling anywhere from $160,000 to $600,000 annually in base salary, with significant bonus packages and benefits on top of it. Heck, no one would retire unless they had to when making that kind of money!

As a result, most GenXers never progressed to the head seat but topped out in a lower role in the C-Suite. Individuals born between 1961 and 1979 are generally categorized as Generation X. Here is the bad news for GenXers in the health care space. There is a strong likelihood the GenXer will get passed over for the CEO role in the coming years as the transformation from a volume-based model to a value-based model will come to fruition.

Why? There is a strong likelihood that GenXers had just enough exposure to the fee-for-service era that we are too jaded to fully understand and pioneer the necessary change to a value-based, patient-centered model. Think about it. The two models are in direct contrast to each other, and experienced health care executives fought the required change that was mandated by the ACA out of basic human nature if nothing else. Everyone resists change. But when the change is a complete threat to everything you have ever been taught in your professional career? Yikes!

It's my belief that many health care organizations will skip the Generation X executive when looking for their leader of the future and look directly to a millennial who grew up knowing only technology, patient-centered care, and how to succeed in a value-based model. No bones in their body to resist the change! In fact, it's quite the opposite. An inherent excitement for being part of the transformation to a more humane model—patient-centered care—exists! Further, millennials are growing up in an environment where creative technological approaches drastically change delivery methods overnight in many industries, and health care delivery is no exception. In fact, health care is at the forefront. Millennials will be much quicker to understand and adopt changes driven by technology than those who were trained in a fee-for-service environment where keeping physicians happy was the main priority of the hospital operator. Millennials are no doubt positioned for success as future health care leaders.

Millennials embrace technological advances that improve health and reduce costs. In contrast, many of the holdover chief executives from the fee-for-service era have fought technological implementation every step of the way as a means to control expenses and appease aging physicians. Aging physicians most often hold the few leadership positions in a hospital and are often uninterested in adapting to new practices in the twilight of their career. In fact, many physicians, whether they admit it or not, were threatened by technology as it would in many cases reduce the need for a physician consult and in turn reduce the doctors earning potential.

I saw this frequently as a CEO when dealing with cardiologists. While they would be impressed with updated technology, until someone taught them how to utilize it, what code to bill, and how much reimbursement they would receive for the procedure, the doctor had little interest in the hospital acquiring and implementing the technology, as without additional revenue being generated, the cardiologist often knew that the test result could eliminate the need for a patient to do a billable consult in his or her office.

In contrast, in my experience, millennial physicians, like the youngest of the GenX physicians, are more likely to be focused on opting for a guaranteed salary and an employed position with 9:00 a.m. to 5:00 p.m. daily hours as opposed to the traditional preference of becoming an independent physician. This has been a welcomed trend for integrated health systems like Kaiser Permanente and Medical Foundations which utilize an employment model and have cash stockpiled to provide guaranteed security to these young doctors.

Millennials have also been raised in a generation where self-management of one's personal health has been entrenched in the fabric of their upbringing. Since the ACA was passed in 2010, the majority of millennials will have no recollection of an era in which fee-for-service was the model, diet and fitness were not a priority, and technology wasn't available at your fingertips 24/7 to assist individuals in making better decisions that impact personal health. All they know is the post-ACA mentality. Now it would be naïve to assume that the culture that will result from the drastic changes mandated by the ACA is complete. Millennials are just young enough that the key cultural trends that emerge—the instant use of healthy technology and the importance of self-responsibility and management of one's health—are likely to be a core component of millennial thinking for their entire lives.

As described above, millennials have only known an iPad, coordinated care, and instant connectivity. From a lifestyle perspective, the impression they will grow up with is technology that enhances their ability to make healthy decisions and better self-manage their own health. As a result, a healthier and more responsible society will evolve, and it is likely that these same individuals will see a rapid rise to leadership positions in the health care space.

CHAPTER 20

Caring for Mom: Tips from the Trade on Caring for Aging Parents and Selecting a Senior Facility

W E HAVE ALL heard it. It's a universal preference. No one wants to go to a nursing home when they get old. And those of us who are middle aged or older have likely had to look at least one of our parents in the eye and promise them we would never put them in a nursing home. Sadly, many of us who made that promise, myself included, had to break that promise years later as a result of either not having financial resources to hire a caretaker or just simply being ignorant to the options available for senior care.

And we have all heard how this issue will continue or grow as the baby boomers continue to retire. Since 2011, more than 10,000 seniors a day have started turning sixty-five years old. It's middle-aged children, however, that often manage care for parents in their later years.

Before giving you a description of the different levels of post-acute care, I want to share a personal story with you. In 2007, my grandmother Wanda Gerken was well into the final chapter of her life. After her husband of more than fifty years had passed, Grandma's memory impairment quickly progressed, and she entered and lived in an assisted living facility near our home. It was a nice three- or four-star facility just walking distance from her favorite restaurant. The truth is that she had progressed to the stage that without support, a four-hundred-yard walk to the restaurant was probably more of an appeasing dream for all of us than a reality. In retrospect, I don't think it ever happened once in the year she lived there.

After a year, the assisted living company advised my family that my grandmother's memory impairment had progressed, and they no longer felt she was safe to live there. Unfortunately, her Alzheimer's disease had progressed to a stage where she was incapable of a conversation or making any decisions on her own. They provided a few examples of her evolving symptoms and associated struggles as a result. In retrospect, it likely meant my parents could no longer afford the facility as it was probably seeking additional dollars per month to pay for the needed additional oversight to keep her safe.

Either way, we found a residential care facility in our hometown owned by a European couple who lived in the house with the residents, both male and female. Then almost a year later, the owners of the group home contacted my mom to advise her that her mother's needs had grown too intensive for them to care for. We were then faced with an inevitable reality, which was placing my grandmother in a skilled nursing facility. In spite of the fact that my mom and her brother had promised their mom that they would never put her in a nursing home, the doctor advised them they had two choices: pay nearly $7,000 a month for a high-level assisted living memory care unit for Grandma or place her in a nursing home with a locked dementia unit. Grandma's monthly social security income was less than $1,500 a month, and among all family members, there were insufficient resources to pay for a specialized memory care assisted living environment. The toughest decision of my mom's life was put before her and her brother, and it required them to break a promise they had made to their mother years prior.

At the time we placed my grandmother in the nursing home in Fullerton, California, I held the position of chief executive officer at what was then called Western Medical Center Anaheim, an acute care hospital. Although it is customary in America that nursing home patients be taken by paramedics to the nearest acute hospital from the nursing home, they can be taken to other nearby hospitals when it has been requested. Thus, I coordinated with the director of nursing at the nursing home with the request that anytime my grandmother needed to be hospitalized, which is often a regular occurrence for nursing home patients, the nursing home would request grandma be taken to Western Medical Center Anaheim. This worked well for a few months as she was hospitalized several times for two to three days at a time for various acute issues. This allowed me to visit with her daily when she was on-site. You can only imagine how well my staff took care of the CEO's grandmother!

About six months after Grandma first moved into the nursing home, I got a call from my mom that my grandmother had been rushed from the nursing home to the nearest hospital. Paramedics almost always rush to the nearest hospital when it's an emergency. As I hung up the phone in my office at the hospital that day, I knew this was it. I had a premonition several months earlier that I did not want my grandmother to die in my hospital. I called my wife and told her to get the kids from wherever they were and to meet me at the hospital.

When we got to the hospital, my mom asked me to join her and her brother for the meeting with the doctor. "Your mom is no longer able to swallow and is choking on food and aspirating, which is why she has had several recent bouts with pneumonia," the doctor said. "We would like to do a swallow evaluation on her. We will need your consent to insert a feeding tube in your mom for a few days while we conduct the swallow evaluation so she can be nourished." The doctor pushed the consent form across the table for my mom to sign.

As my mom reviewed the consent paper, I intervened and told my mom to hold off. Although the decision was that of my mom and her brother and not mine, I wanted to make sure they understood the implications. My mom had also promised her mom that she would never let her live on a feeding tube in a nursing home, a state that many Americans disparagingly refer to as a "vegetable." So I summarized the situation in my own words for my mom and asked the doctor to correct me if I misstated any information.

> "Mom, what I think I just heard is that Grandma is no
> longer able to swallow food on her own, which is why

she has been losing weight and fighting pneumonia off and on. These concerns, along with general lack of nutrition, are causing her to be in an even greater confused state, and on top of that, she has less energy, so she is staying in bed all day and likely to develop pressure sores and a urinary tract infection since she is incontinent.

"Thus, the doctor is asking you to consent to put a tube in her, which you promised her you would never do. So that you are aware, there are two likely results that will come from doing a swallow evaluation:

1) "The evaluation could show that Grandma is able to swallow, and this was just an accident caused by some other issue (which is unlikely).

2) "The test confirms Grandma is unable to swallow and will need a feeding tube inserted in her abdomen for the remainder of her life to be nourished (which is the likely scenario, as the doctors are already almost certain that she cannot swallow and there are several indicating factors that are already present).

"So, Mom, if you sign this paper, the likely result will be that in two days, your next decision will be this:

1) "Grandma lives on a feeding tube in a nursing home without ever leaving bed for the rest of her life, or . . .

2) "You sign another consent form in two days to remove the feeding tube. Essentially, Mom, you will be asked to sign a consent to 'pull the plug' on your mother.

"While it may be easy to consent to sign to put a tube in, the guilt of being asked to sign it out haunts many people who have done it for years after. Grandma wanted to die peacefully. She never wanted to live in a nursing home, and from what I can gather, she is likely halfway home already as she has not been nourished

for several days. So if you choose not to sign it, call
the family and tell them grandma has a few days left."

I had warned my mom that many families reverse decisions in moments like these. Decisions that had been well thought out and discussed by all family members often fall by the wayside in those highly emotional moments. Let's not ignore the fact that the doctor failed to share the likely scenarios with my mom, and had I not intervened, she would likely have been faced with consenting to pull the plug on her mom. While everyone has their own opinion on how situations like these can be handled, my mom and her brother decided against the feeding tube and requested comfort measures for my grandmother.

One positive thing that came out of her final days is that the doctor injected her with some sort of steroid for comfort and strength, and when I visited her with my wife and children the following morning, she was as coherent as I had seen her in several years. Even though all my children were under the age of ten at the time, my wife, Martine, and I explained to the kids before they entered the room that this would be the last time they would ever see their great-grandmother. And although for kids at that age it had always been awkward meeting, loving and understanding an aging senior with memory impairment, who had never been able to engage them in meaningful conversation at any time in their lives, my kids all stepped up that day. God blessed that situation with so much grace as Grandma looked them all in the eye, and they all took their turn giving her a long hug and kiss, and then they waited outside as I said my goodbyes. It was an amazing moment that God created to make that a positive and uplifting experience. On the way home, Martine and I agreed that even if Grandma lived another week (on water alone), the kids would not go back to see her as the final moments and conversations had been so peaceful for all. I felt so blessed.

I shared this story about my grandmother as it will really serve as an example for many of the points that we will make over the next few chapters. It provides a good example of one family's journey in managing their parents' later years in life. I am personally thankful that it ended on a positive note as my grandmother had a few great moments with my kids that day. I was able to spend a few more hours with her the next day before she passed, but I could see in her eyes that she was pleased with the decision my mom and uncle had made. She never wanted to live that way or without her husband of more than fifty years who had already been gone for more than ten years. Even in those incredibly difficult moments, my mom and uncle were able to honor her wishes. And let's end this story on that note. What I believe to be the most important factor in those difficult end-of-life decisions that undoubtedly result in differing opinions of the adult children is this: do your best to honor your parents' desires even when your guilt and emotion may tell you otherwise. It is their life, and they don't want to continue to be a burden on your life as well. Honor your parents.

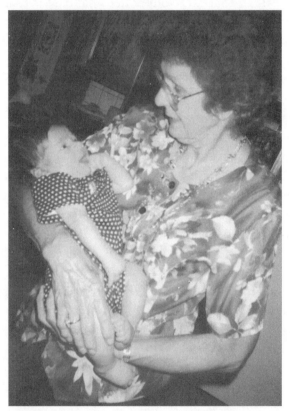

My grandmother Wanda Bell Gerken holds my oldest son after he was born. A few years later, she moved into an assisted living facility.

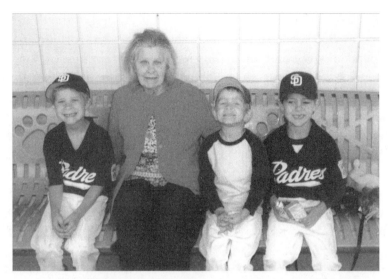

Grandma Wanda with her great-grandchildren. This was one of the days we picked her up from her residential care facility to bring her to watch the grandkids' ball games.

Vetting potential facilities for your loved one:

I want to share one bit of advice for when your doctor gives you the bad news that your loved one is no longer able to live safely on their own. Just like you would for any other important decision in your life, research and shop multiple facilities. Interview the administrator and director of nursing at each facility, as well as the social worker. It's like any other relationship you enter. This could be a long-term relationship with these individuals for you as the family care manager, as well as for your parent. Thus, a good personality fit and finding individuals you are comfortable with is often much more critical than the curb appeal of the facility and which facility has the nicest chandelier in the dining room. Remember, the chandelier does not care for your mom for sixteen hours a day; the people do.

Should I use a care placement adviser?

Care placement advisers can be very helpful in assisting families learn about what needs their loved one may have and which local facilities are best suited to meet that individual's need. Also, they should almost always provide service to you at no charge. They can also serve as an independent voice on each facility's quality, patient satisfaction, and track record. However, that independent decision is almost always being influenced by which facilities are willing to pay them and at what rate (similar to a realtor who may not mention to a buyer that a specific house is for sale because the seller has only offered 1 percent or 2 percent commission instead of the customary 3 percent per agent). So a skilled and experienced care placement adviser has crafted his or her message to new clients in a manner that makes sure the facilities that pay better commission to the care placement adviser will always be positioned best. It always comes back to capitalism, does it not?

Be aware of the manner in which most care placement advisors are compensated. "A Place for Mom" is the most well-known. Care placement advisers are compensated by keeping the first month's rent when your loved one is placed in the facility. This is the other side of the care placement business that your family should be aware of before deciding to work with a care placement adviser. To clarify, the good news is it should not ever cost you anything for this service. The bad news is that the assisted living facility or residential care facility often looks down upon these advisors as they feel they are unnecessary.

This is most common with the larger assisted living companies. They pay expensive marketers and nurse liaisons to visit families in the hospital before discharge and provide tours of the assisted living, so they see no need for a "middle man." However, it is beyond the control of assisted living facilities to prevent care placement advisers from working with clients, so most assisted livings still accept patients from care placement advisers and compensate them as a result, although it would undoubtedly be their preference not to work with care placement advisers. Thus, if your loved one passes away in the initial thirty days of being placed in the facility, the facility in many cases would not be compensated at all as the first month's rent went to the care placement adviser.

Buyer, beware! When you register online for a senior care assistance organization, you are often consenting to them being your sole representative (similar to a realtor). This type of "care placement" organizations, in many instances, can provide families valuable guidance and support in a time that is emotionally, physically, and financially challenging. I have worked professionally with many of these care placement advisers, and they can be an extreme value to families in these times. However, buyer, beware!

The second you enter your personal information on the website (which is prior to them allowing you to navigate off the home page), as soon as you check the box and click enter, they will argue that they are your legal representative (or realtor if you will), and it is difficult to get out of this mess if you end up not electing to use their service. I have heard of cases of these larger companies claiming a year later that when an individual moves into a facility, even if the care placement company never spoke with or assisted the family, the company will claim that the family first discovered the facility on its website, and therefore, they will demand compensation from the facility. Many states are contesting this aggressive business practice used by many of these placement agencies as it is perceived as "predatory."

I have personally heard many assisted living executives refer to care placement advisers as "extortionists," and unfortunately in some cases, they may have an argument. However, so long as you are aware of the business model and practices, care placement advisers can be extremely helpful for individuals managing the next phase of care for aging parents.

Touring prospective facilities

When you go to tour a facility, do not schedule an appointment. Go see the facility when they are unprepared for you to see the reality of the environment. One of the most challenging times of the day for any senior facility is from 7:00 a.m. to 9:00 a.m. as residents are waking up and getting dressed.

One of the saddest realities I experienced in my career as a health care administrator was the lack of family support most nursing home patients receive. While everyone has busy lives, approximately 80 percent of the patients in the nursing homes I managed had less than two visitors a month. The 20 percent who had visitors almost always had daily visits from different family members. It was clear to me that families kept an organized calendar to make sure there was frequent socialization—which is a key factor in maintaining cognitive skills for aging seniors.

Even when Grandma Gerken was institutionalized in her golden years, both at the assisted living and the residential home, while my entire family all lived within a ten-minute drive, her weekly visits were most often one visit or less combined. I am not casting blame but pointing out that I myself have been on both sides of the fence. For most individuals, one of the best means to handle difficult situations, particularly as they relate to parents and grandparents aging, is to limit exposure to the reality of the situation. One of the saddest realities of my life is when I am uncomfortable around an aging or ill loved one who is in the hospital or suffering from memory impairment when I know it's an individual I have spoken to regularly for my entire life. The reality is that it is just plain uncomfortable, and many people handle it by turning the other way as much as possible so they don't have to deal with it as often.

On a closing note, I would try to go by the assisted living and residential home to visit her every Saturday and take her to my kids' soccer, baseball, and basketball games (which I was often coaching). In her younger years, watching her grandkids' games always brought her great joy. During her senior years, there were only a few moments in which I could tell if she was getting any joy out of it at all. In spite of that, I knew for myself, for my children, for my parents, for my grandmother when she returned to health in heaven, and for my God who was always watching, in charge, and leading me through inspiration, that taking Grandma to those games was the right thing to do.

CHAPTER 21

Caring for Mom Part 2: Understanding the Different Levels of Care for Seniors

A S SENIORS AGE, there seems to be a common confusion that arises or graying of the understanding that all levels of senior housing are one and the same—which they are definitely not. There is a distinct difference between a skilled nursing facility and an assisted living facility. And while assisted living facilities can be extremely costly in some markets, there is also the increasingly common option of residential care facilities (often called board and care or group home).

As more and more seniors are impacted by memory impairment, dementia, and Alzheimer's disease, the trend of the aging senior seems to be a lack of understanding in the difference between these levels of care. Rather than hear my grandparents, and now my parents, say in their early retirement years, "please do not ever send me to a *nursing home*," as they age and their cognitive impairment increases, the statement more commonly becomes "please do not ever send me to one of those *senior facilities*." Essentially, this is a last ditch cry to remain in their own home or home environment as an individual's activities of daily living (ADL) and their ability to self-manage diminishes—with or without a living spouse to provide support.

So in reality, there are almost always several key factors working here that lead to seniors preferring not to be "institutionalized" in their golden years. It's important to be aware and consider the emotional and social implications of this decision, not just the physical and memory-based concerns that lead to the need to put a senior in a home.

1. Dignity and human nature being the most prominent. (What senior wants to leave their home, particularly if they lived there for many years?)
2. Finances: Not enough income to cover costs or unwillingness to pay based on limited income.
3. A promise to a deceased spouse.
4. A promise to a living spouse and the guilt that encumbers both when the decision is inevitable.
5. A desire to pass on as a preference over living the rest of life in an institution. This is even truer if they have been widowed and want to "join their spouse."
6. Length of stay: many seniors want to think that the trip to the facility (whether nursing home or assisted living) will be temporary.
7. On the contrary, I believe that the reason many seniors fight the decision to be institutionalized is that they subconsciously understand (as they have seen many friends go through it in prior years) that institutionalization is a key symbolic milestone in the aging process. It often symbolizes the beginning of a rapid decline in health and an individual's ability to perform activities of daily living. Thus, institutionalization is often the first major step before more severe health concerns including advanced Alzheimer's disease, dialysis, feeding tubes, breathing support, palliative care, hospice services, and other undesirable concerns arise. The most severe and final step in the process of course is the ultimate, inevitable outcome—death.

The truth is, the difference between these levels of care is night and day. Assisted living facilities often offer upgraded services for additional fees, including housekeeping services, ADL support, and other amenities and services. I used to joke with my wife all the time, even in my thirties, and say, "This assisted living facility is immaculate. They make all three meals for you, do your dishes, make your bed for you if you request, and have a lounge stocked with our own private wine locker. Let's move in today!" The amenities of assisted living sounds attractive to many young parents when they are in the midst of raising kids or teenagers who, in spite of your best repeated efforts, can't seem to figure out how to clear the table after meals, do dishes, wash their own laundry, or pull two sheets up daily to "make their bed"!

But let's be real here. While most newly built assisted living facilities appear to be four- or five-star resorts that come with monthly price tags ranging from $3,000 to $8,000, nursing homes, on the other hand, fall to the opposite end of the spectrum. Most skilled nursing facilities are aging, with only a few private rooms. And in spite of best efforts to make the facility feel more like a residential care facility, almost everything about a nursing home still looks and feels like a hospital. The reality is that nursing homes are in fact extended hospitals for aging, ill patients with multiple chronic issues. To meet the stringent regulations of operating as a nursing home, it is almost inevitable that the physical plant will look and feel like a hospital no matter how aesthetically pleasing the artwork, furniture, design, and other décor may appear.

The next few pages provide a brief, commonsense description of the different options for senior care, the associated costs with each level, the truth about their quality outcomes, and whether or not I would be willing to send my own mom to receive care. We start with the highest and most intense level of post-acute care and work our way down to the least intrusive and least restrictive means of care which is nonmedical home care.

Long-Term Acute Care Hospital (LTACH)

What is an LTACH? While an LTACH was a thriving business model in the fee-for-service era, the number of LTACH beds will diminish greatly between 2016 and 2020. Not only has the federal government put a moratorium on building new LTACH facilities, but the managed care payment methodologies of the ACA present a significant threat to LTACHs surviving under their current business model. From a consumer perspective, however, an LTACH may appear to look like a nursing home on the exterior, but on the interior, they look almost identical to hospitals. The truth is that they are licensed as hospitals. LTACHs are for clinically complex patients with multiple chronic illnesses. The most common type of patients admitted to LTACH are those in need of a vent or "trach" for breathing support or wound care management (for bed sores or pressure ulcers often developing as a result of poor hydration, malnutrition, and lack of mobility).

Average length of stay: Twenty-five days

Payment options and implications: Medicare and insurers in rare cases will pre-authorize LTACH stays for very sick patients, but only with justification and clinical evidence that the patient could not be adequately cared for at a lower level of care like skilled nursing.

Un-fun fact about LTACH: Dr. Christopher Cox, a critical care specialist at Duke University School of Medicine, told the *New York Times* in June 2014 that in his experience, approximately half of the patients who enter LTACH facilities die within a year, less than 15 percent return to an independent life, and the remainder are placed in custodial care (nursing home or residential care facility) for the rest of their lives. With less than 15 percent returning to an independent life, you can understand why the federal government is continually finding additional means to limit the type of patients that qualify for LTACH and reducing reimbursement as well.[8]

Would I send my mom to LTACH? No, I would not send my mom to an LTACH even if the doctor presented a strong argument for recovery. I would fight to keep my mom in the acute hospital as all the same services are provided. The difference is the acute hospital is incentivized financially to get her well, independent, and back home. The LTACH is financially incentivized to find a way to keep her in their facility for approximately twenty-five days. LTACH is a last resort, and if my doctor was discussing this as an option, I would inquire into hospice services as it is likely your loved one is nearing end of life and their body is giving up on them.

---

[8] 1 New York Times. At These Hospitals, Recovery Is Rare, but Comfort Is Not, Gina Kolata, June 23, 2014.

Acute Rehab Facility

What is an acute rehab facility? An acute rehab facility is a post-acute facility in which patients who need aggressive physical, occupational, and/or speech therapy go to recover after a hospital stay. It is licensed as a hospital and can also tend to many acute clinical conditions. Acute rehab hospitals are similar to nursing homes but can handle sicker patients and are usually a lot nicer aesthetically as to date they have been reimbursed significantly more than nursing homes. One important thing to note about acute rehab is that a patient must be willing to participate in rehab for at least three hours a day, five days a week. Some of that rehab can be while they are sitting down or in bed, but the majority of it cannot. Also, you do not need a hospital stay to go to an acute rehab. You just need a doctor's order, and you can be admitted directly from home.

Average length of stay: Twelve to fifteen days

Payment options and implications: This is a Medicare-covered benefit, and some insurers will pay as well. However, the ACA has led to insurers opting to send you to a nursing home for these services whenever possible as they can most often provide the same rehab services in a nursing home at half the price or sometimes even at a third of the price. Thus, if you are told that you or a loved one needs to go to a nursing home for a few weeks for rehab, ask if acute rehab is an option. You will likely have to aggressively push to get it approved, and they will likely still say no.

Un-fun fact about acute rehab: Acute rehab was created to serve the needs of a small niche of patients who had unique needs or aggressive therapy. Over the years, acute rehab lobbyists were able to show quality results in acute rehab facilities, so more procedures were approved for reimbursement. As Medicare spending spiraled out of control, similar to the situation with LTACH, legislators and insurers alike turned up the heat on acute rehab, with many suggesting that like LTACHs, acute rehab facilities are not necessary. While that is an aggressive stance, acute rehab does provide quality services and is the best approach for a handful of situations, including trauma recovery, traumatic brain injury, amputation, stroke, and a few others. One of the most notable acute rehab hospitals in the country is Craig Hospital in Colorado, and the role of acute rehab facilities that survive the next ten years will be very similar to Craig Hospital's approach—which is to be very good at a few specialized services (and leave the rest of the rehab services to the nursing homes).

Would I send my mom to an acute rehab? Yes. If her insurer is recommending a nursing home for two to three weeks of therapy, I would demand an acute rehab instead. However, I would likely lose that battle if her insurer requires a preauthorization. And if I am going to lose that battle to try and get a preauthorization after serving as an acute rehab CEO and working in the industry for fifteen years, it is likely you will lose that battle as well. We all need to get used to the thought of seniors rehabilitating in a nursing home.

Skilled Nursing Facility (SNF)

What is a skilled nursing facility? SNFs, more commonly known as nursing homes or convalescent homes, provide two levels of care. First, there is custodial care, also called long-term care. Custodial care simply means that the patient will be at the SNF for life as they are unable to live alone. When someone is unable to return home, having clinical needs that cannot be cared for in their own environment, they are in the SNF until they die.

Second, short-term rehab care. These patients recently had an accident (such as a fall) or illness and as a result ended up in the hospital. Once they are recovering in the hospital, the doctor discharges them directly to an SNF to rehabilitate. The goal of the SNF is to get a person healthy and strong enough to function independently at home. The stay is usually two to three weeks for short-term rehab patients. SNFs prefer short-term rehab patients as they are reimbursed at two to three times the daily amount that they receive for long-term care patients.

Average length of stay: Short-term rehab: fourteen to twenty days (although insurers will push for less); long-term care/custodial: life.

Payment options and implications: SNF is a covered benefit for Medicare, Medicaid, and almost all insurers. Insurers will push for a length of stay between seven and ten days in most cases and will authorize additional days only on an as needed basis.

Fun fact about SNF: The length of stay for many SNFs nationally is traditionally twenty days for rehab patients. By no coincidence, Medicare paid for 100 percent of an SNF rehab stay for the first twenty days. The minute patients were advised they had a daily co-pay, they miraculously felt strong enough to return home. What a coincidence! While this twenty-day no-co-pay rule remains in place for some Medicare products, the twenty-day co-pay rule will likely disappear over the next few years as alternative payment models are offering preauthorizations and controlling the length of stay.

Would I send my mom to SNF? If I have a choice, then "no." But the more likely answer is "yes," as I illustrated in the story of my grandma Gerken. In many situations, an SNF may be inevitable. Will she forgive me for it? Not likely.

Assisted Living

What is assisted living? It's a facility built to best meet our seniors' needs who no longer wish to live alone, or are unable to care for themselves. They often do not have any health concerns that would require an SNF, but many assisted living sites accommodate a growing number of health concerns by staffing on-site nurses. Many are very nice and look like five star resorts!

Average length of stay: Forever. Or until their need for care becomes too extensive and the patient needs to transition to an SNF. Or until they run out of money. Believe it or not, running out of money may be the most common reason for a patient to leave. The usual result is the person enrolls in Medicaid, the national health care reimbursement program for individuals without resources (welfare).

Payment options and implications: Assisted living is cash pay. That means your cash. In very few instances will the insurer pay for assisted living days. Although, paying for assisted living days is going to become more common in coming years as effective assisted living care has been proven to reduce medical spending. Thus, if this is an option for you, inquire with your insurer, facility of choice, or care placement manager if there are any options for assisted living coverage or reimbursement.

Un-fun fact about assisted living: Assisted livings in many cases provide as much medical care as a skilled nursing facility. Thus, if you have the money, you can almost always avoid the SNF if you are willing to pay for it. It may be $10,000 a month at the assisted living, but hey, its capitalism and money talks!

Would I send my mom to assisted living? Absolutely. Remember I joked earlier, some days I wish my wife and I could move in as well and have all our meals cooked, room cleaned and dishes done for us!

Memory Care/Dementia Unit

What is a memory care/dementia unit? There are two types of facilities for memory care patients who are a danger to be left unsupervised and in an unlocked facility. The first would be a locked SNF unit. The second would be an assisted living specializing in Alzheimer's disease and memory care. Silverado Senior Care is a national leader in this area. I mention this as they have taken an active role in research both nationally and internationally, and I appreciate them taking a proactive leadership role.

Average length of stay: Forever.

Payment options and implications: Memory care in assisted living is cash pay and is much more expensive than a normal assisted living unit. You can expect to pay in the range of $5,000 to $9,000 a month for these services. In an SNF, reimbursement works the same for the locked unit as it does for a regular SNF bed (it is paid for by Medicare and Medicaid in specific scenarios).

Un-fun fact about memory care/dementia unit: Everything about these units is un-fun. However, it is often the best or only environment of care for when a patient's memory is diminishing. Also, companies like Silverado are doing a fantastic job of implementing modern technology to best meet these patients' needs.

Would I send my mom to memory care/dementia unit? Yes. It may be inevitable if your mom has progressing Alzheimer's disease or dementia.

Residential Care Facility

What is a residential care facility? Same as an assisted living, but it's an actual home in a neighborhood. There are likely several in your community; you just might not know it. They are much more affordable in many cases than assisted living, and many prefer the home environment as an alternative to the hotel atmosphere of an assisted living facility. In many states, a residential care facility can house up to six seniors. In other states, it's up to ten seniors. They are often called board and care.

Average length of stay: Like assisted living, forever or until their needs become too intense for the residential caretakers and need to transition to an SNF. Or until they run out of money. However, very often, an individual can find a residential care home that is inexpensive enough that their monthly social security income or retirement check covers the monthly total.

Payment options and implications: Residential care facilities are cash pay. That means your cash.

Un-fun fact about residential care: There are a lot of shady characters running residential care facilities as there is little oversight by regulatory agencies. Thus, vet them well when you are selecting. This is where a care placement adviser can assist. Also, pop in unannounced often to see what really goes on when you are not there. Many offer remote video monitoring of some sort if the state permits.

Would I send my mom to a residential care facility? Absolutely. But I would vet it well and pop in unannounced often.

Home Health Services

What are home health services? Home health services are medical and rehab services provided in the home. They are most often given after a hospital or nursing home stay to assist an individual in returning to a person's prior level of function, which allows them to independently manage their primary activities of daily living. Care is provided by licensed nurses and therapists.

Average length of service: Six weeks. (Although patients often reenroll in a new episode if there is still a need after the initial six-to-eight-week episode).

Payment options and implications: Home health is a covered benefit for Medicare and most insurers. Similar to SNFs, insurers will seek a shorter length of service, likely ten to fourteen days for initial preauthorization, as opposed to allowing six to eight weeks of service as was the norm under the Medicare benefit in the prior model.

Un-fun fact about home health services: Similar to residential care facilities, there are a lot of shady characters providing home health services as there is little oversight by regulatory agencies, and it is very difficult to monitor home-based care. Thus, vet them well when you are selecting. The federal government is very leery of home health as there is rampant fraud, and it has put a freeze on any new home health agencies opening in several states in recent years as a result.

Would I enroll my mom in home health services? Absolutely. Make sure it's a reputable agency. You don't want any shady characters caring for your parent or stealing her valuables!

Nonmedical Home Care and Private Duty Nursing Services (Home Care)

What is home care? Similar to home health, home care is home-based care that is less expensive than home health and most often for the less-acute patient. The caretakers are often unskilled but may have a minimal amount of training or may be a licensed certified nurse assistant (CNA). The result is that caretakers can stay longer. Home care is popular for families whose aging parent cannot be left alone safely but prefers not to put them in a nursing home. It is very common for individuals with memory impairment issues, whether they live alone or not—they often need constant supervision.

Average length of service: It can be two hours a day or twenty-four hours a day. It can be temporary while the kids or spouse is out of town or at work or long term until a senior passes away.

Payment options and implications: Home care is cash pay. That means your cash. In very few instances will the insurer pay for home care. Although, like assisted living, paying for home care is becoming a more common trend as effective home care has been proven to reduce medical spending. Thus, if this is an option for you, inquire with your insurer, facility of choice, or care placement manager if there are any options for home care coverage or reimbursement.

Un-fun fact about home care: It is often the last days of honoring your promise not to institutionalize your parents. It is the time that reality sets in that within a few months, the caretaker will not be enough, and you will be forced to resign to 24/7 care in an institution.

Would I sign my mom up for home care? Absolutely. It is my first choice. Also, it is important to note that while insurance may cover home health services, those benefits are often capped and limited to a certain number of hours or days, while home care is not subject to those restrictions. That's why paying cash for home care is often a better approach than letting your insurer pay for home health services if the financial resources are available.

Hospice Care

What is hospice care? Specialized end-of-life care and support.

Average length of stay: Most often until death. A small few recover and are removed from the hospice service.

Payment options and implications: Hospice is a covered benefit by Medicare and insurance.

Un-fun fact about hospice: No one wants to be the person who tells a family "your loved one is dying." Thus, the toughest thing about hospice is that it is underutilized as everyone is afraid to advise the patient and family that hospice is the most appropriate option for the patient. Because the doctor, nurse, and caretaker are often scared to advise the patient and family, hospice services oftentimes are underutilized. It's a real bummer because hospice is a great benefit.

Would I sign my mom up for hospice? Absolutely. I would use a reputable agency, not a mom-and-pop.

Palliative Care

What is palliative care? A multidisciplinary approach that focuses on comfort care and reducing pain and discomfort. The goal is to improve the quality of life at the end of life by focusing on relief from pain, symptoms, physical stress, and emotional stress as opposed to focusing on healing and recovery.

Average length of stay: Until death.

Payment options and implications: It is sometimes a covered benefit and sometimes not. You need to ask your insurer. If the insurer is Medicare, ask the hospital discharge planner assigned to your loved one if in fact palliative care is recommended.

Un-fun fact about palliative care: It's largely an untapped resource in many communities as there has not traditionally been reimbursement in place for palliative care. It is different than hospice (as death is not always imminent but the patient prefers not to seek healing treatment), but they are largely confused and discussed in the same manner.

Would I sign my mom up for palliative care? Absolutely.

Adult Day Care

What is adult day care? A community-based facility that cares for seniors during regular business hours. It is often utilized by those who cannot afford a caretaker, a spouse of a patient who still works, or adult children who are caretakers but work during the day.

Average length of stay: Daily, from 8:00 a.m. to 6:00 p.m. in most cases.

Payment options and implications: It is sometimes a covered benefit and sometimes not. You need to ask your insurer. It is oftentimes provided as a community service, or there is available grant money for some individuals. There are also tremendous social benefits for seniors who utilize adult day care as it keeps them engaged both physically and mentally. Without participation in adult day care, it is much more likely that a senior will self-isolate, physically decompensate, and be at higher risk for injury or fall in the home.

Un-fun fact about adult day care: It's largely an untapped resource in many communities as there has not traditionally been significant reimbursement. It is a tremendous benefit for assisting a senior in maintaining his or her fitness and independence.

Would I sign my mom up for adult day care? Definitely.

CHAPTER 22

Long-term Care Insurance?
Medicare Advantage? How Do
I Pay for My Parent's Care?

WELL, THIS MAY be a short chapter as I really do not have an answer for individuals seeking advice on how to best plan and care for parents who are aging and may need access to expensive care. However, I am confident that the one piece of advice I give everyone is critical: go visit with an elder law attorney as soon as you can to begin planning and understanding how reimbursement works.

I took my own advice and went to an elder law attorney with my dad in late 2015. My mother's Alzheimer's disease is progressing, and we went to learn about financial options for her care. I have worked in the industry almost twenty years, and I still learned a lot from this visit. Visiting a lawyer who specialized in long-term care and elder estate planning is a must.

You will be advised on how to manage assets. You will get a better understanding of Medicare being a short-term benefit that is most often only applicable when you are healing or recovering from an illness or injury. Once recovery plateaus, a patient becomes a "custodial" or long-term care patient and is required to pay privately or get Medicaid coverage. You will be reminded that Medicare is a fund that patients paid into for years as employees while they worked. You will also understand that Medicaid is essentially welfare for individuals with limited assets. Medicaid also only covers care in a nursing home. You will be advised of the plusses and minuses of your parents placing their home in a trust. You will be advised that the federal government can look back into finances two to three years prior to Medicaid being approved to see how money was handled and often seek to recover funds from children or simply deny the parent the Medicaid benefit.

You will also learn, perhaps the most surprising thing I learned, that any assets that remain when a Medicaid patient dies, the federal government has first dibs on the amount of money they spent on that individual. To clarify, if your grandmother was on Medicaid for the last two years of her life and Medicaid paid out $200,000 on her care, when she passes away and her home is sold, the federal government could and would legally claim the first $200,000 from the sale to be theirs.

What about long-term care insurance? Should you buy it? The best answer I can give you is that this is a personal decision. If you have the funds to justify it, then it is worth considering. If not, perhaps putting that same money into a savings account will be equally effective. The benefits of having a long-term care policy that I have witnessed working in the industry included coverage of co-payments for skilled (short-stay therapy) days in a nursing home, as well as extended-stay coverage when the patient's primary insurance no longer covered a stay but they were not confident enough to return home yet. Other benefits of long-term care insurance include in-home care coverage for both medical and nonmedical home health services, as well as short-term respite stays in senior institutions for seniors who live with a family while the family is on vacation.

I wish I could be more helpful on this topic. But that's all I got. It's a personal choice.

On the topic of opting for Medicare Advantage instead of maintaining traditional Medicare benefits, there are more data and facts available to families to research to select the best product for your loved one. While many doctors will insist on their patients staying in traditional Medicare fee-for-service, as those doctors retire and the ACA mandates kick in, you will largely see the disappearance of Medicare fee-for-service as we knew it by 2020. With that in mind, the choice of Medicare Advantage becomes simpler: which plan will I choose.

Study the benefits. Some offer dental coverage; some don't. Some offer more lucrative vision benefits; some don't. Some offer two replacements a year for lost dentures, others just one. Some have $0 or $1 co-pay medications; others don't. My best advice is to understand your loved one's greatest needs and select an insurer that best caters to those needs.

And some may ask, "What is a dual plan?" A dual plan means that a health plan (insurer) manages the individual's Medicare and Medicaid benefits. If a Medicare beneficiary has no assets (other than their home) to speak of and has qualified for a Medicaid benefit, they are enrolled in a dual coverage plan. So in addition to having a Medicare benefit (as a result of paying into the fund on every paycheck they ever received), they also have Medicaid benefits (welfare) as they have no other means to access care if it is not a covered Medicare benefit. Operationally, both Medicare Advantage and dual plan enrollees will likely need preauthorization for all services moving forward. Remember, it is becoming a managed care world!

CHAPTER 23

Single-Payer System: Does the ACA Story End with a Single-Payer System?

DOES THE AMERICAN healthcare debate end with a single-payer system? I get this question a lot. Let me first dissect the question. What is a single-payer system? That translates to converting to a government-payer approach. At the rate the costs of health care are growing, with new expenses and more middlemen entering the picture daily, it is not out of the question.

But rather than guess at what we don't know, let's start with what we do know. The government prefers not to be in the medical insurance industry. The ACA pushed more of the government's responsibility to private insurers who have been proven to provide care at a lower cost than government-run programs. Thus, the government was just bankrolling a process that they previously managed, and their track record for managing was not great. So why not just hand a check to the private insurer and say, "This is all you get." If each year you give out just a few dollars less per patient than the prior year, then your costs come down.

In theory, while this model is designed so that the government's costs will come down, the savings have not historically trickled down to the consumer. Insurer profit margins continue to grow in most cases, while the cost of health care to businesses and consumers continues to increase at an alarming rate.

One thing I am absolutely confident in: America is reaching a tipping point on how high a family's or business's medical costs can go before they just opt out and pay cash in emergencies.

Thus, when I get the single-payer question, I always assume it to suggest that costs in health care are rising too fast for the general public and small businesses to keep up. Therefore, the assumption is that the bubble eventually bursts, and the country implements a government-funded single-payer insurance model overnight. This is commonly known as socialized medicine.

Ask Canada how that's going! Waiting months to get on the schedule for an operation can be the norm.

A few factors driving additional costs in health care include aggressive unionization pushes by the clinical staff in hospitals and post-acute facilities. In addition to increasing wages, unions are pushing for patient ratios, which limit the number of patients a single nurse or caretaker can care for. This serves as a double whammy for hospitals whose costs are significantly impacted by each of those factors. As nurses push for more regulation, hospitals incur additional costs and often begin cutting resources that are not mandated, including lower-level caretakers. In turn, nurses grow more frustrated as the caretakers who previously bathed the patients and assisted with bowel movements and other simple tasks are often eliminated by the hospital as they are not required by law—only the nurse is.

Similarly, the unions are pushing aggressive regulatory changes and increases in pay for home-based caretakers as well. In 2015, there was a national movement toward a $15-an-hour minimum wage. In addition, unions are pushing for more scrutiny and increased background checks for home-based caretakers. This all adds up to additional costs to the taxpayer and the family needing care. Until recently, it was not unheard of for a home-based care company to charge only $15 an hour. In 2016, several states approved a $15-an-hour minimum wage that will be implemented incrementally by 2022, and this will inevitably be another contributing factor in the rapid increase of health care costs.

So let's assume we did go the single-payer route. The immediate reaction would be an aggressive growth in the concierge medicine space. Are you familiar with this term? Many of you are familiar, as at some point in the last ten years, you received a letter in the mail from your longtime personal physician who was converting to a concierge medical practice model. The letter likely said something like the following:

> Dear longtime patient and friend,
>
> It has been an honor to care for you and your family for all these years. It is my hope to continue this relationship. However, because my practice has grown so big, I am no longer able to accommodate everyone. Also, due to the rising costs of health care delivery, I am no longer able to keep practicing medicine independently. Thus, I am joining a group called (fill in the blank here).
>
> I wanted to let you know that this group brings an emerging new model in health care. Whether or not you have medical insurance coverage, this group limits the amount of patients that are affiliated with my office. The good news is you have the opportunity to be one of these individuals. Those who join will have an annual fee and can walk into the office any day at any time in addition to scheduling an appointment. Those who don't unfortunately are no longer able to receive care at our office.
>
> Sincerely,
>
> "Your Longtime Doctor"

So to translate what you just read: "For $10,000 a year, I will still be your doctor. Otherwise, I am no longer able to be your doctor. Good luck finding a new doctor that's any good." Welcome to the world of concierge medicine.

In almost every socialized medicine society, you see components of a socialized medicine industry. This is not all that different than plastic surgery in America at present. You can access plastic surgeons via insurance in certain situations, but most plastic surgeons have converted to a cash pay, cosmetic surgery business model.

It's a natural evolution in a society that provides socialized medicine or a single-payer solution. Access becomes more difficult, and the rich find a way to get better care in a shorter amount of time. This is called concierge medicine.

Modern Healthcare magazine reported in February 2016 that the United States ranked first internationally on health care as a percentage of its gross domestic product (GDP), with 16.4 percent. That is a 31.2 percent increase over the last thirteen years, the fifth-largest growth rate internationally,[9] with no end in sight. In fact, the nation with the fastest-growing percentage of health care as a share of GDP is the Netherlands, which uses a two-tiered system (government plus concierge offerings). The three nations who ranked higher in health care share growth for GDP all have single-payer systems.

So to get back to the original question "Will we end up in a single-payer system?" I think it is too difficult to predict at this point. The certainties that we know are that costs are rising at an alarming rate, Americans are retiring at an increasing rate, and costs for families and businesses to access medical coverage are reaching a tipping point. Thus, major reform is necessary and in many ways already under way. It's just too early to tell if it will turn the tide.

So if you want my honest opinion on single payer, here it is: I am unconvinced that single payer will ever be our only option. And even if the decision was made to convert to single payer, it would take several years after the fact to convert as we learned with the unexpected delays and roadblocks incurred during the implementation of the ACA.

---

[9] Modern Healthcare; Page 34, February 8, 2016. "By the Numbers: Healthcare's Share of GDP."

CHAPTER 24

Where Should I Invest in the Health Care Space?

W E SAVED THE funnest chapter until the end! Based on my travels in the last few years and being one of the leading strategists in the post-acute space, I have seen a lot of great new technology. I have seen a lot of good products that did not last and others that gradually became sustainable. Before I tell you which areas I see growing, let's discuss the process of becoming a viable solution in the health care space.

First, stick to the first sales lesson you ever learned. Before you tell someone how to solve their problem, implement the powerful skill of listening by asking what their problem is. So many salespeople approach hospitals, doctors, and insurers and present a concept by opening with "here is how we are going to solve your problem." I cannot tell you how many meetings I was in after the passing of the ACA in which this happened. The presenters rarely started the meeting by asking what it is we were struggling with.

What I learned is that each hospital, doctor, and market is unique. To assume all hospitals have the same pain points is a foolish assumption. Likewise, to assume all hospitals and doctors were going to have a strong reaction to newly implemented financial penalties as a result of the ACA was another foolish assumption. In fact, there were so many new penalty programs that the smartest thing a salesperson could have done was to start by asking (which of these programs concerns your organization the most and why?). So please, ask someone what their problem is before telling them how you plan to solve it!

Next, a good idea is not always a good business model. For example, there are lots of great websites with high traffic that are not viable business models, but they are great concepts. There are plenty of similar comparisons in health care. Focus on a strong business model and the severity of the problem that the product solves. What are the financial implications and to what organization if the problem is not solved?

With those things in mind, here are a few thoughts. Let us start with areas I would *not* be investing in at present. While there are exceptions to every rule, here are some general areas I would likely avoid investing in for now:

- **Hospitals:** Mixed bag. We are going through an identity crisis as hospitals are being forced to become insurers. I would let the dust settle until 2018 before I invest heavily in acute hospitals. Many individual hospitals will go out of business and close. The government is ratcheting back on the financial lifelines it has been throwing these safety net hospitals. It is my opinion that the federal government knows that some hospitals will close, and in many cases, they are okay with that.
- **Long-term acute care:** No way. Run for the hills if they come asking!
- **Acute rehab:** No way. Same as above. The heyday is over.
- **Skilled nursing:** In a worst-case scenario, the heyday of SNF profits (fee-for-service era) is coming to an end, and margins will shrink significantly. Until payment reform evolves, SNFs will be going through a major identity crisis from 2016 to 2020. Hold off on investing until the trade can reinvent itself.
- **Health care software:** If a company is selling software in the medical space and that software in some way needs to correspond with the hospitals electronic medical record, the most important factor to consider is the market position of that software company as it relates to the top EMR providers. To say it kindly, if the software company is not playing in the same sandbox with Big EMR, it is going to be an uphill battle. I can't underscore this enough. If you need more detail on this, just refer to the Big EMR chapter to reflect on how

powerful they are and how easily they get their giant hospital clients to follow their lead. In short, all other technology is a threat to the hospital budget that they believe should all be theirs. Be very careful and do your research before investing in this space.

– **Telehealth and remote monitoring:** Another likely candidate that could turn out to be fool's gold! This might be surprising to many, but let me explain. Telehealth and remote monitoring are being widely accepted and are going to experience explosive growth in the coming years. However, many organizations, both inpatient (hospital or SNF) or outpatient (home or doctor's office), have had an epic struggle implementing the technology. What's the cause of the struggle? For starters, who pays for the expensive equipment? Even those physicians who are willing to use it may not have any financial incentive to invest their own money. Also, there is so much turnover in post-acute care and home-based care that when a caregiver is trained appropriately, they may not have a flexible schedule enough to meet with the patient in need of telehealth. Third, schedules. There are two parties coordinating telehealth services. As you know, it is hard enough to get everyone in one workplace to coordinate schedules, let alone get another workplace to be ready at the same time. Fourth, in the home, it is very difficult as caretakers do not always see the benefit and are not monitored and scheduled to go to different homes on a regular basis. And fifth, it can be quite expensive to buy technology for one patient and leave it in their home, and the return on investment is just not there at present. Too many roadblocks currently add up to me being unwilling to financially invest in this sector at present.

Now here are the areas that I *would* be investing in:

– **Assisted living:** Remember a few basic concepts:

1. No American wants to go to a nursing home.
2. Assisted living is cash pay, so it is paid in advance.
3. No insurance means no preauthorization required.

4. Minimal government regulation (assisted living is regulated by the Department of Social Services and surveyed once every three years; SNFs are regulated by the Department of Health and surveyed at least annually). This is a slam dunk if you confirm the demand and price the rooms appropriately.

–   **Residential care:** See above. Ten thousand Americans are retiring each day. Price points for residential care per month can be as low as $1,000 per resident and as high as $6,000 per resident. If the house is paid for, you have a lucrative business model. When families cannot afford assisted living and are unwilling to place their loved one in an SNF, the answer is a residential care facility.

–   **Home care:** You already learned how many baby boomers are retiring. Many have scarce resources and limited medical benefits, and all of them would prefer to stay home as opposed to being institutionalized in a nursing home or assisted living facility. These factors all add up to a lucrative business model. Note: in 2015, more than $40 million in venture capital was infused into the home care space. Home care is another slam dunk if you invest in the right company.

Many of these companies may be familiar names including AMADA Senior Care, Cambrian, Care at Home, ComforCare, Home Instead, Nurse Next Door, Right at Home, Senior Helpers, 24Hr Homecare and newer players including Honor. Traditional medical home health companies have started venturing into the space to provide more comprehensive care in the home, including Amedisys and Kindred at Home (formerly Gentiva). I always recommend AMADA Senior Care when friends and hospitals are searching for care as I have found their leadership and programs to be the strongest in the industry nationally. If you are a family in need, or a health system in search of a home care partner, AMADA Senior Care would be my first call. After all, I called them to care for my mom which is why I believe in them—I am a customer (#4MyMom&Yours)!

The insurer wins, which in this case is the home care company managing the patients care at home. We have covered this already, right? The government gives them a check, they manage your care effectively and efficiently, and they get to keep the balance. It's a proven formula.

- **Self-management technology (promoting health and personalized medicine):** While I shy away from provider-supported telehealth and remote monitoring technology at present, I am a firm believer that easily adapted technology that assists in and promotes self-management (Fitbits) will continue to experience explosive growth.

- **Home-based technologies:** Again, self-management in the home that does not require a third-party provider. The difference here again is that the person making the purchase decision (consumer) does not need to rely on a third-party provider to get trained and implement on the technology. The buyer is the user.

Now these opinions are only mine, and they are not scientific, so take them for what they are worth. It will be interesting to look back on this chapter in 2020 and again in 2025 and see how close I was! Good luck with investing and caring for your loved ones and your personal health.

CHAPTER 25

Discharge with Dignity: Changing hospital and physician culture to allow patients to be discharged home

IN LATE 2015 I began promoting a discharge methodology that I had been sharing with my university level students since 2012. I originally called this approach "Discharge Home" or "Taking a Home-First Mentality."

In 2016 however, as I consulted hospital CEO's across the country, several prominent executives confided in me that there most significant operational challenge in transforming to value based care was getting the support of their own hospital-based case management staff. And even those executives who felt they had the full support of their case managers were expressing frustration that the journey to taking a "discharge home first" mentality within their hospital was proving to be difficult if not impossible.

As discussed earlier, the incentives of the fee for service-free-for-all led to deep-rooted cultural practices and behaviors between doctors and case managers. The pattern became to discharge patients to institutions such as nursing homes or acute rehab facilities after a hospital stay. Not only did it reduce the liability of the doctor and hospital (should the patient have a fall or unfortunate incident after they were discharged) but it also became the easiest and quickest way to discharge a patient from the hospital. Yes! The path of least resistance became the preference for all involved.

Discharge with Dignity™: The Discharge Planners New Role - Adopt a "Home-first" Mentality

Start from the left side of guide and work your way to the right if a discharge home is not an option

The Financial Impact of Post Acute Referral Patterns for hospitals, ACO's & Bundles

	Home Care	Assisted Living	Transitional Care Visit	Chronic Care Management	Home Health	Hospice Palliative	SNF	Acute Rehab	LTACH
Degree of Financial and Quality Penalty to Discharging Hospital **Start Here**	None	None	Negligible (its less than 10% of the cost of home health – and it covers 30 days as opposed to 6-8 weeks for HH)	Negligible	Nominal (should rarely be ordered in acute OR SNF setting; send Dr./NP to the home for Transitional Care visit to assess need for HH)	None NA	Moderate	Severe (only for specialized needs that can't be met at a SNF)	Severe (LTACH is truly specialized *acute* care, not post acute care)
Discharge Level	FO	FOADH	AHD	ADWCD	ASN		LR	A	A
Patient Financial Responsibility	$	$$	Nominal	Nominal	Nominal	NA	20% after 20 days	Varies	Varies

LR – Last Resort if skilled need (if patient is unsafe to go home with resources)
ASN – Consider as alternative to SNF if skilled need & Home Care not an option
FOAHD – First Option After Discharge Home; Assisted Living can cause delays in hospital discharge; engage AL before discharge

ADWCD – (Order for) All Discharges with Chronic Diseases
A – Avoid unless specialized need; requires physician advisor approval

FO – First Option and consideration for all patients
AHD – (Order for) All Home Discharges

Source: Dr. Josh Luke, www.JoshLuke.org. For permission to use or re-print, please email luke@usc.edu

As time went on, three decades in all, doctors and case managers got much better at justifying why nursing homes were supposedly a "better and safer" option for patients upon discharge than "taking the risk of going home." Their communication and scripting for families and patients got smoother and smoother until they had it down – because every American can't wait to be sent to a convalescent home, errr, nursing home. The reality is that the belief between doctors and case managers that institutionalizing patients on discharge was the more appropriate path for discharging became the accepted norm.

So the patient and family were actually led to feel that by returning home they would be unsafe and potentially at risk...in their own home. That's not just manipulative but extremely powerful when you look at it from a distance, isn't it? Convincing somebody that they are unsafe and at risk in their own home. It seems pretty cavalier on the surface as well.

Combine that with the Federal regulations that ensure Americans have a choice in choosing a post acute facility, and case managers felt empowered to control the process. All they had to do was get patient consent and the path of least resistance became the norm. That's' right, all seniors with Medicare were discharged to a SNF in most cases unless they were educated enough on the laws to challenge the discharge order, the doctor, the case manager and the system as a whole. All in the name of less work, quicker results and the path of least resistance.

In fact, in many situations case managers acted like the "self-proclaimed defenders of patient choice," even bucking hospital administration or anyone who tried to mettle in what they saw as their responsibility and theirs alone. After three decades of this behavior and freedom, the patterns became deep-rooted within most hospitals.

Thus, even those executives that were able to communicate the changing nature of value based care to their case managers in 2016 were contacting me reporting that the behavioral change in discharge planning was either taking way too long or just being road-blocked altogether.

Well, I told you so, didn't I?

That is why as far back as 2012 I developed a guide to help case managers understand two basic concepts:

1.) To encourage doctors and hospitals to consider sending a patient home with resources, so they can age, heal and recover at home (as opposed to in an institution if home is a possibility), and

2.) The guide utilizes multiple colors to illustrate and represent the financial penalties for hospitals and doctors if patients are consistently discharged from the hospital to post-acute institutions (such as acute rehab, long term acute care or skilled nursing).

This guide presents a dramatic shift from the mindset of case managers during the fee for service era. The home-first approach is often met with great trepidation by case managers. Actually, millennial case managers which have only ever known value based care have been quite accepting in most cases. But more experienced case managers who have had the luxury of having complete freedom in how and where they discharged patients on a daily basis for the past thirty years are slower to adapt. It is very evident that the majority of case managers were at least initially uncomfortable with the increased level of scrutiny and accountability on their department, but ultimately trough communication, education and empowerment this transition can take place.

My relationship with case managers as a whole has traditionally been rocky, as when I present I have been known to be provocative. This issue of patient choice, patient steering to select providers, patient and family education, and adopting a home first mentality have been passionate topics of mine since 2010. Why? Because 2010 is the year that my mother was first diagnosed with Alzheimer's Disease. Thus, I was flattered and honored when both the Case Management Society of America and the American Case Management Association both contacted me in 2016 to contract with me to present to their members. In fact, I was the keynote speaker to more than 2,500 case managers at the CMSA Annual meeting in Long Beach, California in 2016 (see photo on page 64).

The most flattering part of that process were the words that the then Executive Director of CMSA shared with me when she first reached-out to me about presenting: "Josh, my members need to hear your message whether or not they like it. And even if you are provocative, it will get them thinking more on the lines of value based care." It was one of the biggest compliments anyone in the industry could give me!

The Discharge with Dignity Guide was introduced to many for the first time in that presentation in Long Beach and it rapidly became a primary topic of conversation within the hospital case management industry. The guide came up in almost every conversation I had with case managers throughout the country for the remainder of 2016.

Although the guide in this book is in black and white, the various colors included in the guide are a critical component. Please visit www. JoshLuke.org to see the actual full color guide. Remember, one of the two objectives in creating the guide was to help case managers and doctors understand that continuing their existing discharge patterns, largely institutionalizing patients after hospitalization, would lead to significant financial penalties. The colors in the guide illustrate these penalties. However, transforming to a home first mentality, and attempting to get patients home to recover if they are able and have access to appropriate resources, should be the goal of each discharge. The Discharge with Dignity Guide illustrates that organizations who successfully transform in this manner will not only receive higher patient satisfaction scores (as patients prefer to go home and not a nursing home), but the organization will reap the financial benefits as well.

Multiple hospitals around the country have called to share with me that they have implemented this guide for daily use. They subsequently share that the financial viability of their ACO's and bundled payment programs have improved, and penalty amounts have come down as well.

All this said, I want to close with one key point. It's all about providing the right care, at the right place, at the right time. No exceptions. However, undoing years of cultural behaviors is a difficult task. The Discharge with Dignity guide has helped several health systems work through this extremely difficult process.

In 2016, I had the pleasure and honor of co-presenting with Amy Bassano to a large group of healthcare executives, Congressman and leaders in Nashville. At the time, Amy Bassano was the Executive Director of the Center for Medicare and MediCaid Innovation. Other than getting to know her, one of the most significant benefits of co-presenting with her was the relationship we were able to develop during the preparation for the presentation. The day of the event I was able to sit with her for an hour and discuss all of these topics with her and it was truly an honor. Even though I kept inviting her objections and challenges to my positions, I was flattered to learn that she had few objections to any of the perspectives shared in this book.

But the one point she made consistently that I share with you today is that each patient is an individual and it would not be prudent to suggest that "all patients should go home from the hospital." That is not at all what the Discharge with Dignity guide is designed to accomplish. The guide is to be used as a tool to change the deep-rooted, long-standing behavior that was in direct contrast to this mentality for many years, which was to discharge the majority of patients from the hospital to an institution.

What's the point? The point is simple: Right Care, Right Place, Right time. But start from a place of trying to get patients home, before considering an institution.

Just imagine that the patient is your mother. Then it becomes easy.

CHAPTER 26

ObamaCare. Trump. So what now?

S O 'THE DONALD' won the election and promised to repeal ObamaCare as one of his first acts. In actuality, Congress beat him to it before he even took office by passing initial repeals in both houses prior to inauguration day. Then, true to his word, just hours after President Trump was inaugurated, he signed an executive order repealing ObamaCare. The order was very generic, clearly a political statement and deferred many decisions on how to roll-back specific initiatives in the ACA to Congress or the state level.

Let me ask you something. Who do you think the most surprised person in the country was on election night? Well I would guess it was Donald Trump. Several media outlets even suggested that he acknowledged this fact!

With that in mind, there were very few transition plans in place when Trump was elected. Other than an ACA repeal, it was the great unknown. With that in mind, how can we as individuals and organizations begin to prepare for the unraveling of the Affordable Care Act?

First, the early 2017 declaration of ObamaCare being dead on arrival was more ceremonial than factual. Even after the GOP raised its hands in victory and declared Obamacare dead, the public initially saw and felt very little impact.

After the declaration of death, the GOP began to pick apart individual mandates and pieces of healthcare legislation to begin addressing them individually. The truth is that several components of the ACA were failing so miserably that even if the Democrats were in control, changes would have needed to be made early in 2017. For example, in many states the insurance exchanges were already failing miserably prior to the election.

So how does this impact you? What about your business or employer?

The reality is both personally and professionally you are unlikely to be impacted in 2017 and 2018 by much change as a result of healthcare reform. Trump's first two Cabinet nominees for healthcare, Tom Price and Seema Verma, both came with a track record of crossing the aisle when needed to gain consensus and get results. But these results will take time.

Unfortunately, as stated earlier in the book, increased premiums are more likely than a decrease in the near future. From a consumer standpoint, it is unlikely the undoing of ObamaCare will lead to a decrease in your monthly family health insurance premium. Although there is no evidence to date that premiums will continue to increase, that would be a more likely option than a reduction.

Why? Well for one it is capitalism, and with change brings added expense. Historically any new added expenses for the insurer are inflated and passed onto the consumer. Unless insurers are able to find operational efficiencies that allow reduced costs in other areas, an increase in premiums remains more likely than a decrease in 2018. Any increase you experience in 2017 will not likely be as a result of the ACA repeal.

Not convinced? Lets take a brief look back at recent history. The two primary consumer goals of ObamaCare were increased access and affordability. While the ACA unquestionably increased access, this expansion in coverage was done largely at the expense of those already insured – middle and upper class American's. While access expanded as a result of the ACA, costs skyrocketed for many. It was a prime example of the re-distribution of wealth in America that was a staple of the Obama era. In fact, in many cases family health costs reached a tipping point to which families opted-out of health insurance altogether.

Myself included for a short time. My wife and I made a calculated decision to go without health insurance in 2013 when I was between jobs. Many have a story similar to mine – pay premiums in excess of $1,000 a month, or roll the dice and your family goes without.

President Trump is a free-enterprise capitalist before all else, so expect that everything he pushes will start with a pro-business mindset. Thus, any restrictions that the ACA placed on businesses, both small and large, will be analyzed and scrutinized. Look for more flexibility for employers to provide coverage for employees, including tax or payroll deduction incentives and increased access to health savings accounts.

Expect that the max contributions for health savings accounts will be increased, and that money left over annually can then be taxed and collected by the individual – a change from most health savings plans of the past. It is also widely anticipated that other changes will be made to the health savings account that provide greater flexibility and thus serve as an incentive for higher participation.

There is talk of age-adjusted tax credits for healthcare that will allow individuals to save money to shop on the open market for their plan of choice. There were several GOP plans circulating in early 2017 supporting increased control at the state level for managing MediCaid funds, allowing more flexibility to local government and business.

Also, expect a flurry of non-traditional options and technologies including telehealth and remote monitoring expansion to be offered that can improve your health. However, the evolution to self-managed healthy lifestyles and wellness comes with a restriction: self-management.

The majority of the technological advances that bring efficiency to the delivery system require a commitment from the individual. That commitment could be time, effort, investment or simply learning a technology. Think Fit Bit, iPad, calorie counting applications or simply logging into the individual patient portal that is used by your hospital. The ugly beast known as accountability! We can't count on others to keep us healthy. Thus, caring for oneself and technology become more critical – an area where millennials clearly have the advantage! While millennials no doubt feel picked on at times, there is no doubt they are more prepared for the incoming trends in healthcare delivery – which are rooted in technology and self-management.

Without self-management or a caretaker that makes the commitment to learn, improved community health and increased cost efficiencies in care delivery will continue to plague the industry.

If you are one of the individuals who did get coverage as a result of the Affordable Care Act, it is likely you will still be able to access some type of program through your state, as Congress is likely to give much more control to each state in managing its own Medicaid funds. What is yet to be seen is whether or not you will have a choice in selecting your carrier. As discussed earlier, with or without the ACA, the Obama Era made access to healthcare a much higher priority in American society as a whole.

One thing that Trump, Price, and Verma are all unified on is deferring to the states to figure out how they spend their own money, which should be very welcome in most states as HealthCare has proven to be so local and so unique in each market. Although this delegation of Medicaid funds and decision making may ultimately squeeze existing MediCaid funds out of more populous states like California, there seems to be significant support for this approach amongst Trump's appointee's.

So will you still have access to coverage? Probably. Will it be more expensive? Maybe, as Seema Verma is known to emphasize self-responsibility (financial), or an attempt to apply for employment as a condition for coverage. For a lot of providers that translates to less revenue as the lower class, even when required by law to make co-payments for care, is more often than not unable to secure the resources to cover the co-payment for services.

The talk within the Beltway in early 2017 was largely focused on 'universal access' to insurance for Americans as opposed to 'mandated coverage'. In theory, this should bring overall costs down nationally. But theories are often proven wrong in capitalism, now aren't they?

ObamaCare may be dead, but Americans need for access to affordable care is not.

With that, I will sign off by saying that I would appreciate any feedback you are willing to offer on this book. You can look me up on LinkedIn or Twitter @JoshLuke4Health or @ExAcuteTheBook. Thanks again for caring enough to read to the end! I thoroughly hope you enjoyed this book and I appreciate anyone who is willing to take a few minutes and share their thoughts by doing a book review on Amazon. The entire process takes about three minutes:

1.) Go to Amazon.com
2.) Type "Ex-Acute 2017" in the search box and click on "Ex-Acute 2017 in books"
3.) Click on the book image
4.) Click on "Submit a review of this book"

Thank you for your continued support, and if you need a speaker to present to your business, sales team, trade organization, church group or any other audience that you think could benefit, I would love to come present, entertain and educate your group on how to keep healthcare affordable and still get access to the best doctors and hospitals! Until next time!

GLOSSARY

Affordable Care Act (ACA): The Patient Protection and Affordable Care Act (PPACA), commonly called the Affordable Care Act (ACA) or, colloquially, Obamacare, is a United States federal statute signed into law by President Barack Obama on March 23, 2010. Together with the Health Care and Education Reconciliation Act, it represents the most significant regulatory overhaul of the U.S. health care system since the passage of Medicare and Medicaid in 1965. Under this act, hospitals and primary physicians would transform their practices financially, technologically, and clinically to drive better health outcomes, lower costs, and improve their methods of distribution and accessibility. (Definition source: Wikipedia, March 2016)

Alternative payment models (APM): A term used to describe new health care reimbursement programs designed by the federal government for the Medicare program as a part of the Affordable Care Act. In 2016, there were two reimbursement methodologies considered to be APMs: accountable care organizations (ACO) and bundled payment programs. (Definition source: Josh Luke, February 2016)

Accountable care organization (ACO): A health care organization characterized by a payment and care delivery model that seeks to tie provider reimbursements to quality metrics and reductions in the total cost of care for an assigned population of patients. A group of coordinated health care providers forms an ACO, which then provides care to a group of patients. The ACO may use a range of payment models with asymmetric or symmetric shared savings, etc. The ACO is accountable to the patients and the third-party payer for the quality, appropriateness, and efficiency of the health care provided. According to CMS, an ACO is "an organization of health care providers that agrees to be accountable for the quality, cost, and overall care of Medicare beneficiaries who are enrolled in the traditional fee-for-service program who are assigned to it." (Definition source: Wikipedia, March 2016)

Bundled payment for care improvement (bundled payment program): Defined as the reimbursement of health care providers (such as hospitals and physicians) "on the basis of expected costs for clinically-defined episodes of care." Unlike fee-for-service, bundled payment discourages unnecessary care, encourages coordination across providers, and potentially improves quality. In a bundle, a set amount of money is allocated for the entire episode. If the amount exceeds the allocated total, then the initiator (manager) of the bundled payment program does not receive additional dollars for the care. If the episode of care ends up being less than the allotted amount, then the initiator gets to keep the savings as profit. (Definition source: Wikipedia, March 2016)

Centers for Medicare & Medicaid Services (CMS): The federal agency, formerly the Health Care Financing Administration, which administers the Medicare, Medicaid, and Child Health Insurance programs. (Definition source: CMS.gov, March 2016).

Discharge with Dignity: Discharge with Dignity is the name of a guide or chart developed by author Josh Luke to be used as a tool for hospital case managers, discharge planners and social workers. In this book a black and white version of the guide can be found on page 145. However, the actual guide utilizes multiple colors to illustrate and represent the financial penalties for hospitals and doctors if patients are consistently discharged from the hospital to post-acute institutions such as acute rehab, long term acute care or skilled nursing. The full color guide is available at www.JoshLuke.org. Hospitals around the country have implemented this guide for daily use as it presents a dramatic shift from the mindset of discharge planners during the fee for service era.

Electronic medical record (EMR): Sometimes referred to as electronic health record or (EHR). EMR refers to computerized medical records and order entry by physicians and caretakers. Because health care providers were slow to implement technology, the Affordable Care Act mandated the implementation of EMR by both hospitals and doctors (see "Meaningful Use" below). (Definition source: Josh Luke, March 2016)

Emergency department doctor/physician: A doctor who consults patients in the emergency department. Emergency department physicians do not operate a private practice. Their sole job is to care for patients while they are in the emergency department of a hospital. For example, if you go to the hospital, your family doctor will not consult you in the emergency room. An emergency doctor, who was trained in emergency medicine, will care for you.

Fee-for-service (FFS): Fee-for-service reimbursement is the primary methodology that the federal government utilized to reimburse doctors and providers for delivering health care services for approximately fifty years in the United States until the passing of the Affordable Care Act in 2010. Doctors and providers are paid an individual payment for each service rendered. As a result, there is a financial incentive to doctors and providers to order additional services. (Definition source: Josh Luke, March 2016)

Health and Human Services (HHS): The U.S. Department of Health and Human Services (HHS) is the U.S. government's principal agency for protecting the health of all Americans and providing essential human services, especially for those who are least able to help themselves. The mission of HHS is to enhance the health and well-being of Americans by providing effective health and human services and by fostering sound, sustained advances in the sciences underlying medicine, public health, and social services. (Definition source: Grants.gov, March 2016)

Hospitalist: A doctor who consults patients in the hospital. Hospitalists do not operate a private practice. Their sole job is to care for patients while they are in the hospital. For example, if you go to the hospital, your family doctor will most often not go to the hospital to care for you. Thus, a hospitalist, usually an internal medicine doctor, will care for you while you are a hospital inpatient.

Meaningful use: Meaningful use sets specific objectives that eligible professionals (EPs) and hospitals must achieve to qualify for CMS incentive programs. Meaningful use is using certified electronic health record (EHR) technology to (1) improve quality, safety, and efficiency and reduce health disparities; (2) engage patients and family; (3) improve care coordination, population, and public health; and (4) maintain privacy and security of patient health information. Ultimately, it is hoped that the meaningful use compliance will result in better clinical outcomes, improved population health outcomes, increased transparency and efficiency, empowered individuals, and more robust research data on health systems. (Definition Source: HealthIT.gov, March 2016)

Medicaid: Medicaid is a federal and state-run insurance program, similar to welfare, for those individuals and families at or below the poverty line (Definition source: Josh Luke, March 2016).

Medicare: Medicare is a federal insurance program for Americans over the age of sixty-five (Definition source: Josh Luke, March 2016).

Medicare Advantage: Medicare Advantage plans, sometimes called Part C or MA plans, are offered by private companies approved by Medicare. If you join a Medicare Advantage plan, you still have Medicare. You'll get your Medicare Part A (hospital insurance) and Medicare Part B (medical insurance) coverage from the Medicare Advantage plan and not the original Medicare. Medicare Advantage plans cover all Medicare services. They may also offer extra coverage. Medicare pays a fixed amount for your care each month to the companies offering Medicare Advantage plans. These companies must follow rules set by Medicare. However, each Medicare Advantage plan can charge different out-of-pocket costs and have different rules for how you get services. These rules can change each year. (Definition source: Medicare.gov, March 2016).

Triple aim of health care: As introduced by former CMS director Don Berwick, it is summarized as (1) a healthier population, (2) improved medical care, and (3) reduced costs and inefficiencies in delivering care. His first book, *Readmission Prevention: Solutions Across the Provider Continuum*, was the top selling health care book of 2015.

ABOUT THE AUTHOR

Josh Luke, Ph.D., is a motivational speaker, acclaimed internationally for his educational, motivational and often humorous presentations. He is a social media influencer and has been called by many "The Voice of American Healthcare" for his bold and poignant predictions that one-by-one came to fruition for hospitals and doctors dating back to 2011. His willingness to discuss publicly what others preferred left unsaid in healthcare is one of the many reasons he was featured in a Huffington Post feature article in 2016.

The route that led Josh to become a leader in Healthcare Reform is both poignant and inspirational. By the age of 26, he accomplished his early career dreams of working in sports marketing with some of the biggest names in the world of sports, a position that would be envied by many. Then, at an age when other young people are still trying to figure out their path in life, Josh made a drastic course correction in his career. Listening to his heart, and seeing the drastic need to be a voice for the unheard, Josh was called to action by the declining health and onset of Alzheimer's disease of both his maternal and paternal grandmothers. Josh shares some of the heart wrenching stories of his family's journey through caring for an aging loved one, as well examples of the emotional and financial struggles and choices made not just by his family, but by so many Americans in today's world.

In this book, you will read Josh's story about the exact moment he made the decision to dedicate his time and energies to serving in the health care sector, rapidly rising through the ranks of health care administration, and becoming one of the country's youngest hospital CEOs by the age of 32. There simply is no one else with the vast knowledge and experience necessary to author this book, and provide critical information to those seeking care for their loved one, be it an aging parent, or simply caring for a child.

After learning in 2010 of his own mother's diagnosis with Alzheimer's disease at age 65, a time when most American's begin to consider retirement and their golden years, Josh became a vocal advocate for Alzheimer's research. In 2015 alone, he donated more than $25,000 to the Alzheimer's cause and continues to contribute to fight the disease.

With a rich teaching history in public policy and Healthcare Administration at numerous universities, Josh most recently designed healthcare course work for the University of Southern California's *Sol Price School of Public Policy*. He also dedicates time each year to being active in health care advocacy in our government, and Josh now shares his experience, knowledge and inspiration worldwide.

His first book was the top selling health care book of 2015.